Bone Circulation Disorders

Guest Editors

MICHAEL A. MONT, MD
LYNNE C. JONES, PhD

ORTHOPEDIC CLINICS
OF NORTH AMERICA

www.orthopedic.theclinics.com

April 2009 • Volume 40 • Number 2

SAUNDERS an imprint of ELSEVIER, Inc.

W.B. SAUNDERS COMPANY

A Division of Elsevier Inc.

1600 John F. Kennedy Blvd. ● Suite 1800 ● Philadelphia, PA 19103-2899.

http://www.orthopedic.theclinics.com

ORTHOPEDIC CLINICS OF NORTH AMERICA Volume 40, Number 2
April 2009 ISSN 0030-5898, ISBN-10: 1-4377-0515-4, ISBN-13: 978-1-4377-0515-7

Editor: Debora Dellapena

Orthopedic Clinics of North America (ISSN 0030-5898) is published quarterly (For Post Office use only: Volume 40 issue 2 of 4) by Elsevier Inc., 360 Park Avenue South, New York, NY 10010-1710. Months of publication are January, April, July, and October. Business and Editorial Offices: 1600 John F. Kennedy Blvd., Suite 1800, Philadelphia, PA 19103-2899. Customer Service Office: 6277 Sea Harbor Drive, Orlando, FL 33887-4800. Periodicals postage paid at New York, NY and additional mailing offices. Subscription prices are $244.00 per year for (US individuals), $424.00 per year for (US institutions), $288.00 per year (Canadian individuals), $508.00 per year (Canadian institutions), $355.00 per year (international individuals), $508.00 per year (international institutions), $122.00 per year (US students), $177.00 per year (Canadian and international students). Foreign air speed delivery is included in all *Clinics* subscription prices. All prices are subject to change without notice. **POSTMASTER:** Send address changes to *Orthopedic Clinics of North America*, Elsevier Periodicals Customer Service, 11830 Westline Industrial Drive, St. Louis, MO 63146. Customer Service (orders, claims, online, change of address): Elsevier Periodicals Customer Service, 11830 Westline Industrial Drive, St. Louis, MO 63146. Tel: 1-800-654-2452 (U.S. and Canada); 314-453-7041 (outside U.S. and Canada). Fax: 314-453-5170. E-mail: journalscustomerservice-usa@elsevier.com (for print support); journalsonlinesupport-usa@elsevier.com (for online support).

Reprints. For copies of 100 or more, of articles in this publication, please contact the Commercial Reprints Department, Elsevier Inc., 360 Park Avenue South, New York, NY 10010-1710. Tel.: 212-633-3812; Fax: 212-462-1935; Email: reprints@elsevier.com.

Orthopedic Clinics of North America is covered in *MEDLINE/PubMed (Index Medicus), Cinahl, Excerpta Medica,* and *Cumulative Index to Nursing and Allied Health Literature.*

Printed and bound by CPI Group (UK) Ltd, Croydon, CR0 4YY

Transferred to Digital Print 2011

Contributors

GUEST EDITORS

MICHAEL A. MONT, MD
Director, Rubin Institute for Advanced
Orthopedics, Center for Joint Preservation
and Reconstruction, Sinai Hospital of
Baltimore, Baltimore, Maryland

LYNNE C. JONES, PhD
Associate Professor, Orthopaedic Surgery,
Johns Hopkins Orthopaedics at Good
Samaritan Hospital, Baltimore, Maryland

AUTHORS

ROY K. AARON, MD
Professor, Department of Orthopaedics,
The Warren Alpert Medical School of Brown
University, Providence, Rhode Island

NICHOLAS AIGNER, MD
Consultant, Orthopedic Hospital Vienna
Speising, Speisingerstrasse, Vienna, Austria

MUHAMMAD AJMAL, MD
Orthopaedic Staff, Department of Orthopaedic
Surgery, Veterans Affairs Hospital, Nashville,
Affiliated with Vanderbilt University, Nashville,
Tennessee

HARLAN C. AMSTUTZ, MD
Medical Director, Joint Replacement Institute
at St. Vincent Medical Center, Los Angeles,
California

TAKASHI ATSUMI, MD, PhD
Professor and Chief, Department of
Orthopaedic Surgery, Showa University
Fujigaoka Hospital, Showa University School
of Medicine, Yokohama, Japan

DOUGLAS BALLON, PhD
Associate Professor, Citigroup Biomedical
Imaging Center, Weill Medical College of
Cornell University, New York, New York

STEPHAN BECKER, MD
Consultant, Orthopedic Hospital Vienna
Speising, Speisingerstrasse, Vienna, Austria

PETER M. BONUTTI, MD
Director, Bonutti Clinic, Effingham, Illinois

EDWARD Y. CHENG, MD
Professor of Orthopaedic Surgery; Mairs
Family Professor, Department of Orthopaedic
Surgery, University of Minnesota, Minneapolis,
Minnesota

DEBORAH McK. CIOMBOR, PhD
Associate Professor, Department of
Orthopaedics, The Warren Alpert Medical
School of Brown University, Providence,
Rhode Island

JONATHAN P. DYKE, PhD
Assistant Professor, Citigroup Biomedical
Imaging Center, Weill Medical College of
Cornell University, New York, New York

FRANK J. FRASSICA, MD
Robert A. Robinson Professor of Orthopaedic
Surgery; Department Chair, Johns Hopkins
University School of Medicine, Baltimore,
Maryland

VALÉRIE GANGJI, MD, PhD
Associate Professor, Department of
Rheumatology and Physical Medicine, Erasme
University Hospital, Université Libre de
Bruxelles, Bruxelles, Belgium

JEAN WM. GARDENIERS, MD, PhD
Department of Orthopaedics, Radboud
University Nijmegen Medical Centre,
Nijmegen, The Netherlands

ROBIN N. GOYTIA, MD
Orthopedic Fellow, Johns Hopkins
Orthopaedics at Good Samaritan Hospital,
Baltimore, Maryland; Fondren Orthopedic
Group, Texas Orthopedic Hospital, Texas

JEAN-PHILIPPE HAUZEUR, MD, PhD
Professor, Department of Rheumatology,
Centre Hospitalier Universitaire de Liege
Sart Tilman, Belgium

DAVID S. HUNGERFORD, MD
Professor, Department of Orthopaedic
Surgery, Johns Hopkins Orthopaedics at Good
Samaritan Hospital, Baltimore, Maryland

MARC W. HUNGERFORD, MD
Assistant Professor, Department of
Orthopaedic Surgery, Johns Hopkins
Orthopaedics at Good Samaritan Hospital,
Baltimore, Maryland

LYNNE C. JONES, PhD
Associate Professor, Orthopaedic Surgery,
Johns Hopkins Orthopaedics at Good
Samaritan Hospital, Baltimore, Maryland

TOSHIHISA KAJIWARA, MD, PhD
Clinical Assistant Professor, Department
of Orthopaedic Surgery, Showa University
Fujigaoka Hospital, Showa University School
of Medicine, Yokohama, Japan

HARPAL S. KHANUJA, MD
Fellowship Director; Assistant Professor,
Department of Orthopaedic Surgery, Johns
Hopkins Orthopaedics at Good Samaritan
Hospital, Baltimore, Maryland

HEE JOONG KIM, MD
Professor, Department of Orthopaedic
Surgery, Seoul National University College
of Medicine, Seoul National University
Hospital, Seoul, Korea

KYUNG-HOI KOO, MD
Professor, Department of Orthopaedic
Surgery, Seoul National University College
of Medicine, Seoul, Korea

MICHAEL KUSKOWSKI, PhD
Clinical Psychologist, Minneapolis Veterans
Affairs Medical Center, Minneapolis,
Minnesota

NANETTE LAMEIJN, MD
Department of Orthopaedics, Radboud
University Nijmegen Medical Centre,
Nijmegen, The Netherlands

FRANZ LANDSIEDL, MD
Head of Department, Orthopedic Hospital
Vienna Speising, Speisingerstrasse, Vienna,
Austria

DAWN M. LaPORTE, MD
Assistant Professor; Residency Program
Director, Johns Hopkins University School
of Medicine, Baltimore, Maryland

MICHEL J. LE DUFF, MA
Joint Replacement Institute at St. Vincent
Medical Center, Los Angeles, California

JONATHAN H. LEE, MD
Chief Resident, Department of Orthopaedic
Surgery, Columbia University, College of
Physicians and Surgeons, Columbia University
Medical Center, New York, New York

YOUNG-KYUN LEE, MD
Fellow, Department of Orthopaedic Surgery,
Seoul National University Bundang Hospital,
Seongnam, Korea

AKIHIKO MAEDA, MD, PhD
Assistant Professor, Department
of Orthopaedic Surgery, Showa University
Fujigaoka Hospital, Showa University School
of Medicine, Yokohama, Japan

DAVID R. MARKER, BS
Medical Student, The Johns Hopkins
University School of Medicine, Baltimore,
Maryland

A.J. MATAS, MD
Professor of Surgery, Department of Surgery,
University of Minnesota, Minneapolis, Minnesota

MIKE S. McGRATH, MD
Fellow, Center for Joint Preservation and
Reconstruction, Rubin Institute for Advanced
Orthopedics, Sinai Hospital of Baltimore,
Baltimore, Maryland

ELIZABETH MEIZER, MD
Registrar, Orthopedic Hospital Vienna
Speising, Speisingerstrasse, Vienna, Austria

ROLAND MEIZER, MD
Registrar, Orthopedic Hospital Vienna
Speising, Speisingerstrasse, Vienna,
Austria

DOMINIK MERANER, MD
Head of Department, Orthopedic Hospital
Vienna Speising, Speisingerstrasse, Vienna,
Austria

BYUNG WOO MIN, MD
Professor, Department of Orthopaedic
Surgery, Keimyung University, School of
Medicine, Dongsan Medical Center, Daegu,
Korea

MICHAEL A. MONT, MD
Director, Rubin Institute for Advanced
Orthopedics, Center for Joint Preservation
and Reconstruction, Sinai Hospital of
Baltimore, Baltimore, Maryland

RYO NAKANISHI, MD, PhD
Assistant Professor, Department of
Orthopaedic Surgery, Showa University
Fujigaoka Hospital, Showa University School
of Medicine, Yokohama, Japan

WIM HC. RIJNEN, MD
Department of Orthopaedics, Radboud
University Nijmegen Medical Centre,
Nijmegen, The Netherlands

ANDREW SALAMA, DDS, MD
Associate Professor of Medicine, Blood and
Marrow Transplantation Program, University
of Maryland Greenebaum Cancer Center,
Baltimore, Maryland

B. WILLEM SCHREURS, MD, PhD
Department of Orthopaedics, Radboud
University Nijmegen Medical Centre,
Nijmegen, The Netherlands

THORSTEN M. SEYLER, MD
Physician Scientist Resident, Department of
Orthopaedic Surgery, Wake Forest University
School of Medicine, Winston-Salem, North
Carolina

SATOSHI TAMAOKI, MD, PhD
Assistant Professor, Department of
Orthopaedic Surgery, Showa University
Fujigaoka Hospital, Showa University School of
Medicine, Yokohama, Japan

GLENN TUNG, MD
Professor, Department of Radiology, The
Warren Alpert Medical School of Brown
University, Rhode Island Hospital, Providence,
Rhode Island

JEONG JOON YOO, MD
Assistant Professor, Department of
Orthopaedic Surgery, Seoul National
University College of Medicine, Seoul National
University Hospital, Seoul, Korea

KANG SUP YOON, MD
Professor, Department of Orthopaedic
Surgery, Seoul Municipal Boramae Hospital,
Seoul National University College of Medicine,
Seoul, Korea

MICHAEL G. ZYWIEL, MD
Fellow, Center for Joint Preservation and
Reconstruction, Rubin Institute for Advanced
Orthopedics, Sinai Hospital of Baltimore,
Baltimore, Maryland

Contents

Preface   **xiii**

Michael A. Mont and Lynne C. Jones

Outcome Measures for Evaluation of Treatments for Osteonecrosis   **179**

Lynne C. Jones, Marc W. Hungerford, Harpal S. Khanuja, and David S. Hungerford

> With the advent of cell-based therapies, biologics, and pharmaceuticals for the potential treatment of osteonecrosis, it is important to conduct evaluations using scientifically accepted outcomes measures. For the treatment of osteonecrosis, most studies have focused on pain relief, surgery, or the need for surgery, disease progression (advancing stage), and change in lesion size. Quantification of imaging techniques continue to gain in sophistication but have not yet been validated for use in clinical trials. Despite recent interest in using biomarkers or genetic markers in the diagnosis and analysis of disease progression, more research is needed to determine the sensitivity and specificity of these techniques with respect to osteonecrosis.

Osteonecrosis of the Knee: A Review of Three Disorders   **193**

Michael G. Zywiel, Mike S. McGrath, Thorsten M. Seyler, David R. Marker, Peter M. Bonutti, and Michael A. Mont

> Osteonecrosis of the knee is a debilitating disease that is poorly understood. Originally described as a single disorder, it encompasses three distinct conditions: spontaneous osteonecrosis of the knee (SPONK), secondary osteonecrosis of the knee, and post-arthroscopic osteonecrosis of the knee. This article reviews the current knowledge of these distinct conditions by describing their etiology, pathology, and pathogenesis, as well as their clinical and radiographic presentations. The various treatment options available for each condition are reviewed, with a discussion of their rationale and indications, and a summary of results with various techniques. A thorough understanding of these conditions and their distinguishing features is critical to selecting the best treatment option for an individual patient.

Cellular-Based Therapy for Osteonecrosis   **213**

Valérie Gangji and Jean-Philippe Hauzeur

> This review article describes bone remodeling in the context of osteonecrosis as a bone disease, the use of stem cells in bone and vascular diseases, and cellular therapy in osteonecrosis.

Bisphosphonates and Osteonecrosis: Potential Treatment or Serious Complication?   **223**

Robin N. Goytia, Andrew Salama, and Harpal S. Khanuja

> They are commonly used to treat osteoporosis and other diseases that involve osteoclast-mediated bone resorption, including Paget's disease and multiple myeloma. Their use in treating osteonecrosis of the femoral head has been studied and theoretically holds promise. There are complications associated with these medications, however, including the development of osteonecrosis in the jaw.

**Does Statin Usage Reduce the Risk of Corticosteroid-Related Osteonecrosis
in Renal Transplant Population?**   235

Muhammad Ajmal, A.J. Matas, Michael Kuskowski, and Edward Y. Cheng

The relationship between corticosteroids and osteonecrosis is well known. Limited data suggest that statins modulate cholesterol metabolism and may protect against osteonecrosis. The authors analyzed their prospective renal transplant database to determine if statin usage reduces the incidence of corticosteroid-related osteonecrosis and identified 2,881 renal transplantation patients who met the entry criteria. Among 338 patients on statins, 15 (4.4%) developed osteonecrosis, versus 180 of 2,543 (7%) patients who were not on statins. Osteonecrosis-free survival was similar in patients with and without statin exposure.

Bone Marrow Edema Syndrome in Postpartal Women: Treatment with Iloprost   241

Nicholas Aigner, Roland Meizer, Dominik Meraner, Stephan Becker, Elizabeth Meizer,
and Franz Landsiedl

Bone marrow edema syndrome of the femoral head in pregnant women is a rare disease resulting in disabling coxalgia, beginning in the last 3 months of pregnancy and persisting for several months after parturition. The parenteral administration of the vasoactive drug iloprost constitutes a new approach to the treatment of painful bone marrow edema syndrome of the hip of pregnant women. Six postpartal women (8 hips) with bone marrow edema syndrome of the femoral head were treated with iloprost followed by 3 weeks of partial weight-bearing. Relief from pain, restoration of functional capacity, and normalization of the MRI signal pattern were rapidly achieved, thus avoiding the need for surgical intervention. As the substance is contraindicated in pregnancy, therapy may begin only some days after parturition, with a short discontinuation in breastfeeding.

Assessment of Bone Perfusion with Contrast-Enhanced Magnetic Resonance Imaging   249

Jonathan H. Lee, Jonathan P. Dyke, Douglas Ballon, Deborah McK. Ciombor, Glenn Tung,
and Roy K. Aaron

Osteoarthritis and avascular necrosis are common clinical entities with unknown origins. Recently, vascular changes were implicated in the pathogenesis of both conditions. This article discusses the use of novel noninvasive imaging techniques as a means of assessing bone perfusion and quantifying differences seen in osteoarthritis and avascular necrosis. Review of our human data suggests that the MRI contrast dye is retained for longer periods of time, suggesting decreased perfusion out of regions of osteoarthritis and avascular necrosis. Use of such a noninvasive measure of assessing bone perfusion could be useful in the diagnosis, prevention, and treatment of not only osteoarthritis and avascular necrosis but also other entities that affect the musculoskeletal system.

Collapsed Subchondral Fatigue Fracture of the Femoral Head   259

Young-Kyun Lee, Jeong Joon Yoo, Kyung-Hoi Koo, Kang Sup Yoon, Byung Woo Min,
and Hee Joong Kim

Several etiologies can lead to a subchondral fracture of the femoral head, which may result in femoral head collapse and degenerative change. This article evaluates the follow-up results of subchondral fatigue fractures of the femoral head in which femoral head collapse occurred. The study shows that collapsed subchondral fatigue fractures of the femoral head have a benign clinical course quite unlike that of collapsed osteonecrosis of the femoral head.

Respherical Contour with Medial Collapsed Femoral Head Necrosis After High-Degree Posterior Rotational Osteotomy in Young Patients with Extensive Necrosis   267

Takashi Atsumi, Toshihisa Kajiwara, Satoshi Tamaoki, Akihiko Maeda, and Ryo Nakanishi

Osteonecrosis of the femoral head often occurs in patients under the age of 50 years. In this study, the authors evaluated the effectiveness of high-degree posterior rotation in terms of regaining the spherical contour of severely collapsed necrotic femoral head that was moved medially. They also investigated whether or not subchondral fracture disappeared on the medial femoral head on postoperative anteroposterior radiographs as a result of remodeling after this procedure.

Current Status of Hemi-Resurfacing Arthroplasty for Osteonecrosis of the Hip: A 27-Year Experience   275

Harlan C. Amstutz and Michel J. Le Duff

The purpose of the study discussed in this article is to review the authors' long-term experience with this procedure, compare their clinical results to those of other centers, particularly regarding the difficulty of predicting pain relief, and determine the role of hemi-resurfacing in the future.

Outcome of Uncemented Primary Femoral Stems for Treatment of Femoral Head Osteonecrosis   283

Marc W. Hungerford, David S. Hungerford, and Lynne C. Jones

Cementless total hip replacement has been advocated for patients with osteonecrosis of the femoral head. This study examined the outcome of the femoral stem of four generations of an uncemented, proximally porous-coated, chrome-cobalt total hip prosthesis. There were 158 cases in 141 osteonecrosis patients (74 men, 67 women) who had a mean age of 46 years (range, 17–83 years). The mean follow-up was 103 months (range, 20–235 months). The femoral components of 144 cases were not revised and had a mean Harris hip score of 84 ($\pm$15) at final follow-up. Of the 14 revisions (8.9%), the primary reasons for revision were loosening or significant osteolysis. There were one infection and one chronic dislocation. Proximally porous-coated, anatomic, press-fit stems provide excellent long-term results in patients with osteonecrosis of the femoral head.

Total Hip Arthroplasty After Failed Treatment for Osteonecrosis of the Femoral Head   291

Wim HC. Rijnen, Nanette Lameijn, B. Willem Schreurs, and Jean WM. Gardeniers

This article presents results for total hip arthroplasty after failed transtrochanteric rotational osteotomy according to Sugioka and after failed bone impaction grafting, both initially performed for osteonecrosis of the femoral head. After a minimal follow-up of 2 years, 33 hips were studied. In total hip arthroplasty after failed osteotomy, when compared with total hip arthroplasty after failed bone impaction grafting, clinical and radiologic outcome was less favorable, more complications were observed, and there was a higher revision rate for a technically more demanding procedure.

Current Literature: An Educational Tool to Study Osteonecrosis for the Orthopaedic In-Training Examination?   299

David R. Marker, Michael A. Mont, Thorsten M. Seyler, Dawn M. LaPorte, and Frank J. Frassica

Osteonecrosis (ON) of the knee is a debilitating disease that is poorly understood. Originally described as a single disorder, it encompasses three distinct conditions: spontaneous ON of the knee, secondary ON of the knee, and postar-throscopic ON of the knee. This article reviews the current knowledge of these distinct conditions by describing their etiology, pathology, and pathogenesis in addition to their clinical and radiographic presentations. The various treatment options available for each condition are reviewed, with a discussion of their ratio-nale and indications and a summary of results with various techniques. A thor-ough understanding of these conditions and their distinguishing features is critical to selecting the best treatment option for an individual patient.

Index   **305**

Orthopedic Clinics of North America

FORTHCOMING ISSUES

July 2009

The Anterior Approach for Hip Reconstruction
Paul E. Beaulé, MD, FRCSC,
and Thierry Judet, MD,
Guest Editors

October 2009

Minimally Invasive Surgery in Orthopedics
Nicola Maffulli, MD, *Guest Editor*

RECENT ISSUES

January 2009

Spine Oncology
Rakesh Donthineni, MD, MBA, and
Onder Ofluoglu, MD, *Guest Editors*

October 2008

Shoulder Trauma
George S. Athwal, MD, FRCSC,
Guest Editor

July 2008

Patellofemoral Arthritis
Wayne B. Leadbetter, MD,
Guest Editor

THE CLINICS ARE NOW AVAILABLE ONLINE!

Access your subscription at:
www.theclinics.com

Preface

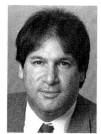 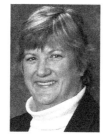

Michael A. Mont, MD   Lynne C. Jones, PhD
Guest Editors

This special issue of *Orthopedic Clinics of North America* represents selected articles from the Fourteenth International Symposium on Bone Circulation. This was a biennial meeting of the Association Research Circulation Osseous (ARCO) that met in Baltimore, Maryland, from September 14–16, 2007.

The goals of the ARCO organization are to update the knowledge base concerning bone circulation and angiogenesis as relevant to clinical practice. The ARCO group meets every other year and conducts a two-and-a-half-day symposium on bone circulation. The program chair and meeting organizer was Lynne C. Jones, PhD. A fine selection of free papers (abstracts of which are to be published in JBJS-Br Orthopaedic Proceedings) was presented by authors from a wide range of countries (including Japan, South Korea, Austria, Egypt, China, United Kingdom, the Netherlands, Belgium, and Germany). Various eminent guest speakers contributed further to the success of the symposium and have manuscripts in this issue. On the third day, Professor David S. Hungerford led a current concepts discussion concerning diagnoses and treatment of osteonecrosis of the hip and future collaborative goals and opportunities.

This issue encompasses a compilation of 13 manuscripts selected from over 40 review lectures and presentations at the Baltimore meeting. The material ranges across many different disciplines dealing with bone circulation and osteonecrosis. This multidisciplinary approach is reflected in articles ranging from basis science to clinical outcomes. We believe that this represents a nice summary of many of the latest principles and the state of the art concerning bone circulation and osteonecrosis.

We would also like to acknowledge certain individuals who were crucial to this meeting, including Deborah Ross, who helped in planning and arranging the symposium. Thank you to Colleen Kazmarek for her invaluable assistance in editing the manuscripts. We would also like to thank various sponsors, including Exachtech (Gainesville, Florida); Ortho Partners, LLC (Richmond, Virginia); Orthopedic Sciences, Inc. (Seal Beach, California); Wright Medical Technologies (Arlington, Tennessee); and Zimmer (Warsaw, Indiana).

For more information, as well as information about future meetings of ARCO, please visit the Web site at www.arco-intl.org.

Michael A. Mont, MD
Rubin Institute for Advanced Orthopedics
Center for Joint Preservation and Reconstruction
Sinai Hospital of Baltimore
2401 West Belvedere Avenue
Baltimore, MD 21215

Lynne C. Jones, PhD
Orthopaedic Surgery
Johns Hopkins Orthopaedics
at Good Samaritan Hospital
Suite 201 GSH POB
5601 Loch Raven Blvd.
Baltimore, MD 21239

E-mail addresses:
rhondamont@aol.com (M.A. Mont)
ljones3@jhmi.edu (L.C. Jones)

doi:10.1016/j.ocl.2009.02.006

orthopedic.theclinics.com

Outcome Measures for Evaluation of Treatments for Osteonecrosis

Lynne C. Jones, PhD*, Marc W. Hungerford, MD,
Harpal S. Khanuja, MD, David S. Hungerford, MD

KEYWORDS

- Treatment outcome • Pain measurement
- Function assessment • Quality-of-life measures
- Radiographic progression

New treatment modalities for osteonecrosis are currently being explored regarding cell-based therapies, biologics, and pharmaceuticals. The ability to evaluate the efficacy and effectiveness of these treatments is contingent upon the selection of adequate outcome measures. Most outcome measures evaluating the treatment of osteonecrosis have focused on the following: clinical performance (pain, function), radiographic progression, surgery or the need for surgical intervention, lesion size, new imaging techniques, or biomarkers.[1] When examining treatments that affect bone, there are certain inherent difficulties in selecting an appropriate outcome measure to determine whether a specific treatment is effective or efficacious. Clinical trials should use validated and medically accepted outcome measures. Outcome measures may be influenced by investigator bias as well as the investigator's knowledge and experience. The variability between patients concerning self-assessment may also hinder the ability to distinguish between effective and noneffective treatment modalities. The use of outcome measures has been complicated by the lack of uniformity in how these tools are applied and interpreted.

A distinction needs to be made between clinical and biologic improvement in response to a specific treatment for osteonecrosis. Clinical improvement relates to pain relief and function restoration and ultimately the prevention or delay of total joint arthroplasty, but it may also include slowing down the rate of progression of the disease. Biologic improvement encompasses decreasing lesion size or increasing bone density or blood flow in a specific area. Although clinical improvement is necessary before a treatment will be accepted by the orthopedic community as a viable therapy, biologic improvement may indicate that the treatment being evaluated shows promise and may yield improved results with optimization (eg, alternative dosing).

This article reviews outcome measures commonly used today in osteonecrosis research and describes additional evaluation methods that may prove useful in the evaluation of new therapies for the treatment of osteonecrosis in the future. This overview also discusses areas of consensus that should be developed to compare the results of different research centers.

OUTCOMES FOR CLINICAL PERFORMANCE

Improvements in pain and function are primary outcomes from the physician's and patient's perspective. With respect to pain assessment, global and localized pain assessments can be made. Function can refer to the quantification of motion or the ability to perform certain tasks. Most commonly, numerical rating scales or visual analogue scales are used. **Box 1** lists several outcome instruments that have been used to assess the hip. **Table 1** provides a summary of outcome measures that have been used for the evaluation of various treatments for early stage osteonecrosis.

Department of Orthopaedic Surgery, Johns Hopkins Orthopaedics at Good Samaritan Hospital, 5601 Loch Raven Boulevard, Suite 201, GSH POB, Baltimore, MD 21239, USA
* Corresponding author.
E-mail address: ljones3@jhmi.edu (L.C. Jones).

Orthop Clin N Am 40 (2009) 179–191
doi:10.1016/j.ocl.2008.10.005
0030-5898/08/$ – see front matter © 2009 Elsevier Inc. All rights reserved.

orthopedic.theclinics.com

Box 1
Patient outcome instruments

Generic

EuroQol[68]

Medical Outcomes Study Short Form-36[7]

Nottingham Health Profile[69]

Visual Analog Scale[70]

Disease-specific

AAOS Hip & Knee and Lower Limb Outcome Forms[6]

Arthritis Impact Measurement Scale[71]

Harris Hip Score[3]

Health Assessment Questionnaire[72]

Lequesne Hip and Knee Indices[73]

McMaster-Toronto Arthritis Patient Function Preference Questionnaire[74]

Merle d'Aubigné & Postel score[4]

Oxford Hip Score[75]

UCLA Activity Scale[76]

WOMAC[5]

Pain Relief

It is assumed that the treatment will bring about pain relief. Any treatment that does not diminish pain, even if it slows down the progression of the disease, will be perceived by the patient as a failure. Much has been written about the measurement of pain in clinical studies, indicating the difficulty of quantifying such as a subjective outcome.[2] It is important to distinguish between pain at rest and pain on weight bearing, because many osteonecrosis patients have indicated that there is an acute onset of pain especially with activity. Several pain scales have been described, such as the McGill Pain Questionnaire and Activities of Daily Living Pain Scale.[2] Many composite scoring systems, both general and disease specific, incorporate a pain subsection. For example, pain is assigned a maximum of 44 points out of a 100-point scale on the Harris Hip Score and a maximum of 6 points out of an 18-point scale for the Merle d'Aubigné & Postel scoring system.[3,4] Questions concerning pain can also be found in the AAOS Hip & Knee Form, the Short Form-36, and the WOMAC.[5–7]

The measurement of pain relief is highly subjective, and studies that use some measure of pain relief are frequently plagued with an inability to show statistically significant differences.

Individuals vary in their threshold to pain and in their ability to detect improvements in pain (sensitivity to treatment).[8] Inclusion of both patient and physician outcome measures of pain may provide some insight into this dilemma. Many studies, particularly with pharmaceutical treatment, have shown a high placebo effect.[9] In other words, control groups may also demonstrate a substantial improvement. Pain may also be influenced by alterations in gait and weight bearing that may have been a consequence of the disease (learned behavior). Furthermore, many patients with osteonecrosis have additional comorbidities that may affect their ability to perceive pain relief.

Function

Several approaches can be used to assess function. Questionnaires may be used as well as direct measures of mobility. According to Meenan and Pincus,[10] functional status reflects the performance of individual tasks. The evaluation may include physician assessment, patient assessment, or the direct observation of specific tasks such as how long it takes to walk 50 feet. Physician appraisals may focus on functional tasks such as range of motion or strength testing, whereas patient assessments may relate to the ability to perform activities of daily living or to perform certain generalized activities.

Many studies evaluating treatment for osteonecrosis have used the Harris Hip Score or the Merle d'Aubigné & Postel score to obtain some appreciation for the level of disability or impairment of function associated with this disease. The Harris Hip Score[3] allocates a maximum of 47 points to functional activities out of 100 total points, whereas the Merle d'Aubigné & Postel Score includes a maximum of 6 points for mobility and 6 points for the ability to walk (total possible score of 18).[4] Function is also incorporated into validated instruments assessing quality of life such as the Short Form-36 or the WOMAC.[5,7]

Although functional scoring is frequently viewed as less subjective than pain relief, this may not always be true. For example, although a patient may be able to flex or extend their hip to an appreciable level, they may not be able to perform certain activities to their level of expectation. Expectations may vary from being able to perform certain activities of daily living to returning to high-impact sports activities. The expectations may be higher for the osteonecrosis population because they are generally younger and more active than patients with other musculoskeletal diseases affecting the hip or knee (eg, osteoarthritis).

Composite Scoring Systems

A number of composite scoring systems have been developed for the assessment of musculoskeletal outcomes.[3,4,6,11,12] As mentioned previously, these systems may be general or disease specific. Because osteonecrosis most frequently involves the hip, composite scoring systems such as the Harris Hip Score[3] and Merle d'Aubigné & Postel Score[4] have been used extensively as a measure of outcome for studies evaluating treatment modalities.

Using the total score as a quantitative measure of clinical performance may actually be less informative than evaluating the subsections for pain or function. Issues may include a lack of justification for the weighting applied to certain categories, a lack of linearity, a lack of clarity relating to certain responses, and the variability of application by the physician. By combining multiple patient attributes such as pain intensity, function, and range of motion into a single categorical judgment, it becomes difficult to make comparisons between different outcome measures used in different studies.[13] Several investigators further categorize the results into excellent, good, fair, and poor. Excellent results may be overreported, reflecting a ceiling effect. Poor is easily defined as an unsuccessful procedure, although there is frequently debate on what is meant by success or failure.

Quality of Life Measures

Although there has been an increased awareness of the utility of patient perspective and outcome measures, this is not a new approach. Prior assessment tools have included the Lee Index, the Convery Index, the Functional Status Index, and others.[2] The two most commonly used quality of life tools in orthopedic research have been the Western Ontario and McMaster Universities (WOMAC) Osteoarthritis Index introduced in 1982 and the Short Form-36 introduced in the early 1990s.[7] The WOMAC has been weighted more heavily for activity limitation, whereas the Short Form-36 is weighted toward assessment of impairment.[14] The WOMAC is a disease-specific instrument, whereas the Short Form-36 is more generalized. Both tools have been extensively validated, although not specifically for osteonecrosis.

Radiographic Progression

Many studies concerning the treatment of osteonecrosis have used disease progression as an outcome measure. Progression has usually been defined as advancement in the stage of disease. Several staging/classification systems have been used, including, but not limited to, the Ficat and Arlet,[15,16] University of Pennsylvania,[17,18] ARCO,[19] Japanese Orthopaedic Association,[20] and Marcus, Enneking, and Massam systems.[21,22] Two outstanding reviews have compared the different classification systems.[18,23]

The diversity of the classification systems used has made it difficult to compare the results of many of these studies. It has been suggested that there are certain radiographic features common to most of the classification systems, such as a sclerotic lesion, crescent sign, head depression, or acetabular involvement.[24] If a consensus could be reached on the collection of specific radiographic characteristics, the data could be entered into any of the classification systems.

Even with this information, there is considerable intra- and interobserver variability in the use of any of the systems. Several studies have shown significant variability when using the Ficat and Arlet, ARCO, and University of Pennsylvania classification systems.[25–27] These studies indicate a lack of agreement in detecting some of the cardinal features of this disease, that is, the crescent sign, flattening of the articular surface, and the beginning of arthrosis. For studies selecting only cases that have not advanced to subchondral collapse, the investigators must show that they can reproducibly identify subchondral collapse. This collapse is one of the most difficult pathologic features to detect on radiographs, as shown by Plakseychuk and colleagues.[25] There are two limitations of the studies concerning the variability of classification: (1) they used radiographs only, and (2) not all of the observers had significant experience in diagnosing nontraumatic osteonecrosis. MRI may be the best radiologic tool to use for distinguishing specific features relating to the staging of osteonecrosis. For example, the crescent sign is easily distinguishable. Furthermore, to decrease the amount of variability within a clinical trial, the interpretation of the scans should be made by one individual with significant experience in this area.

A new method using CT scanning with a helical scanner has been shown to identify more subchondral fractures than MRI or radiography.[28] Stevens and colleagues were able to show 18 of 19 subchondral fractures at 6 months and 20 of 20 fractures at 1 year. The fracture was easy to visualize and well defined. Although CT scanning may not be feasible or necessary for clinical practice, it may be of value in clinical trials.

Surgery Versus the Need for Surgery

Several studies concerning the treatment of osteonecrosis have used "undergoing total hip

Table 1
Evaluation of treatments for osteonecrosis

Study	Treatment	Outcome Measure	Classification System
Stulberg et al., 1991[77]	Core decompression	Harris Hip Score Radiographic progression	Ficat & Arlet
Fairbank et al., 1994[78]	Core decompression	Radiographic progression (radiographs) Need for THR Merle d'Aubigné & Postel hip score	Ficat & Arlet
Koo et al., 1995[79]	Core decompression	Pain–Merle d'Aubigné & Postel hip score Collapse Index of necrosis (MRI)	Steinberg
Kane et al., 1996[80]	Vascularized fibular grafting	Pain THR	Ficat & Arlet
Chang et al., 1997[81]	Core decompression	Pain Radiographic progression THR	Steinberg
Mazieres et al., 1997[82]	Core decompression	Radiologic stage Histologic stage Symptoms	Ficat
Mont et al., 1997[83]	Core decompression	Harris Hip Score THR or poor Harris Hip Score	Ficat & Arlet
Powell et al., 1997[84]	Core decompression	Harris Hip Score Need for THR	Ficat & Arlet
Iorio et al., 1998[85]	Core decompression	Pain Radiographic progression THR	Ficat & Arlet
Scully et al., 1998[86]	Core decompression Vascularized fibular graft	THR	Ficat & Arlet
Wirtz et al., 1998[87]	Core decompression	Merle d'Aubigné & Postel hip score Radiographic progression	ARCO
Bozic et al., 1999[88]	Core decompression	Performance of subsequent operation Radiographic failure (progression to Ficat & Arlet stage III with collapse)	Ficat & Arlet; Steinberg

Study	Treatment	Outcome measures	Classification
Chen et al., 2000[89]	Core decompression	Radiographic progression Severe pain THR	Ficat & Arlet
Maniwa et al., 2000[90]	Core decompression with and without bone graft	Merle d'Aubigné & Postel hip score Radiographic progression THR	Ficat & Arlet
Specchiulli, 2000[91]	Core decompression	Pain Radiographic progression THR	Ficat
Yoon et al., 2001[92]	Core decompression	Radiographic progression THR	Ficat
Aigner et al., 2002[93]	Core decompression	Radiographic progression Harris Hip Score THR	
Hernigou et al., 2002[94]	Autologous bone marrow grafting	THR Harris Hip Score Radiographic progression	Steinberg
Gangji et al., 2004[95]	Autologous bone marrow grafting	Pain–Lequesne Pain–WOMAC Radiographic (radiographs & MRI) progression (with collapse)	ARCO
Lieberman et al., 2004[96]	Core decompression with bone graft and BMP	Pain Radiographic progression WOMAC THR	Ficat & Arlet
Agarwala et al., 2005[97]	Alendronate treatment	THR Clinical parameters (form not cited) Pain–Visual Analog Scale Radiographic (radiographs & MRI) deteriorization	Ficat & Arlet Mitchell
Bellot et al., 2005[98]	Core decompression	Merle d'Aubigné & Postel hip score Radiographic progression THR	ARCO

(continued on next page)

Table 1
(continued)

Study	Treatment	Outcome Measure	Classification System
Lai et al., 2005[99]	Alendronate treatment	THR–based on radiographs (although MRI also done) Need for THR	Steinberg (University of Pennsylvania)
Tsao et al., 2005[100]	Tantalum rod	Harris Hip Score Short Form-12 THR	Steinberg
Ha et al., 2006[101]	Core decompression	Merle d'Aubigné & Postel hip score Radiographic progression of femoral head collapse modified Kerboul angle	Ficat
Neumayr et al., 2006[102]	Core decompression Physical therapy	Harris Hip Score THR	Steinberg
Nishii et al., 2006[103]	Alendronate treatment	Biochemical markers Femoral head collapse (radiographs) Merle d'Aubigné & Postel hip score	ARCO
Veillette et al., 2006[104]	Tantalum rod	Harris Hip Score Radiographic progression THR	Steinberg
Shuler et al., 2007[105]	Tantalum rod	Harris Hip Score THR	Steinberg (University of Pennsylvania)
Song et al., 2007[106]	Core decompression	Harris Hip Score Radiographic progression Any additional surgery	Ficat

Abbreviations: BMP, bone morphogenetic protein; THR, total hip replacement.

replacement" as the distinction between the success and failure of a treatment. This event is a clear-cut endpoint and is used frequently in retrospective studies; however, surgery in and of itself is not an ideal outcome. The "need for surgery" is better. Although surgery may be the end result, the surgery may have been delayed by 2 or more years for various reasons. For example, a patient who has undergone a procedure associated with a notable level of morbidity (resurfacing, light-bulb procedure, vascularized fibular graft) may hold off having a second significant procedure such as a total joint replacement. The patient's health may also preclude the scheduling of a second procedure. When performing survival analysis, the time to diagnosis of an advanced stage needing surgery and not the date of surgery may be more appropriate.[29]

In any study of the treatment of osteonecrosis, time period selection is vitally important. Some evidence suggests that, once diagnosed, significant progression will occur by 12 months.[30] The disease is likely to progress to the point of requiring surgery within 2 years; therefore, any study involving pharmacologic treatment should include a 1-year time period, whereas a 2-year time period may be more clinically relevant. From a pragmatic point of view, if there is no detectable change following treatment by 1 year, it is unlikely that the 2-year effect will be meaningful. One of the challenges in using the classification of "surgery/need for surgery" is that if you select a very early stage of disease and a very short time period, the patient's disease may have progressed significantly but surgery might not yet be indicated; therefore, you have designed your study to preclude ever seeing the outcome that was selected. Furthermore, a treatment may be effective in slowing down the progression of the disease. Depending on the risk-to-benefit ratio as determined by the morbidity of the treatment under study as well as alternative treatments appropriate for the specific stage of the disease, this delay in surgery/need for surgery may be considered a success of treatment. The medical community needs to establish what is considered a meaningful delay (eg, 3, 5, or greater than 5 years).

Complications and Risk—Benefit

Clinic trials routinely evaluate the frequency and morbidity of complications also known as adverse events. The FDA defines an adverse event as any undesirable experience associated with the use of a medical product in a patient. Serious adverse events include death or life-threatening events, hospitalization (acute or prolonged), disability, congenital anomaly, or requires intervention to prevent permanent impairment or damage. However, various treatments for osteonecrosis may also have non-serious adverse events, such as self-limiting fever, indigestion, or mild depression. Non-serious adverse events are frequently overlooked and under-reported.

All treatments should have some assessment of risk—benefit ratio. General factors that may influence the risk of intervention may include patient age, activity level, or heath status (including comorbidities). Disease-specific risk factors may include size of the lesion, stage of the disease (eg, is there evidence of depression or acetabular involvement), or quality of bone stock. Clinical benefit involves pain relief and restoration of mobility and function. However, this must be viewed in the context of duration of relief of symptoms or time of delay for the need for surgical intervention.

Selecting a Clinical Outcome Measure

The choice of outcome tool to use depends on whether you are trying to incorporate its use in your clinical practice or whether you are participating in a clinical trial. Much has been written about using validated instruments, but reliability and responsiveness are equally important. Validity is defined as "a measure of the extent to which an assessment technique measures that which is intended."[2,5] Reliability is the repeatability or the ability of the instrument to measure something consistently.[31] Responsiveness is the sensitivity to change.[2,5] With respect to validity, there are four types: face, content, construct, and criterion.[2,5] Although the majority of outcome measures discussed have been validated,[5,6,31–33] it is important to know which type of validation has been conducted. For further discussion, the reader is referred to several excellent reviews on this topic.[5,13,14,31,34,35]

POTENTIAL OUTCOME MEASURES FOR BIOLOGIC ASSESSMENT
Imaging

Change in lesion size

Lesion size has been shown to be a diagnostic predictor of the success of treatment for osteonecrosis.[36–39] Radiography and MRI have been used to determine lesion size. Due to the differences in methodology, it has been shown that MRI is more accurate in the assessment of lesion size than radiography.[40] This finding is somewhat patently obvious as lesion size determination based on radiography involves multiplying or adding together the measurements from two two-dimensional images, whereas MRI uses several cuts through the region of interest and can more precisely measure the three-dimensional aspect of the lesion. Whether this difference has any impact on the ability to determine at what point collapse is inevitable remains to be proven.

Debate continues on the level of sophistication needed for determining the lesion size reproducibly and accurately. Several investigators have used fairly sophisticated software to evaluate the volume of osteonecrotic lesions.[41] Because it is unlikely that we need the precision to be at a level of cubic microns or smaller, it is possible that simple software packages would still yield useful information. Steinberg and colleagues[42] have described a simple methodology of using tracings from MRI (anteroposterior and lateral) and have found this to be more accurate than using radiography. They argue against the use of the extent of the lesion as described by Koo and Kim.[43] It is also possible that the volume may be less important than the extent of surface involvement. The measurements of Koo and colleagues are related to surface area and may prove to be the better predictor in the long run.

Clinical trials relating to osteonecrosis may incorporate a more sophisticated analysis of lesion size than what has been commonly used in clinical practice. As stated previously, a decrease in the size of the lesion, even though it may not lead to a delay in the need for surgery, may indicate that a treatment has potential and that further refinement of the dose and dosing schedule may be needed to optimize its effectiveness. A recent publication by Takao and colleagues[44] demonstrates that image registration is useful in comparing scans from the same individual and may pick up changes that would not necessarily be picked up with standard methodology. Image registration is a computational process that enables the investigator to align serial images. This technique is more sensitive to detecting small changes in lesion size. Using this technology, the investigators were able to detect a size reduction varying from 2 to 6.5 cm^3.

Bone densitometry

Newer biologic or pharmacologic treatments aim to promote healing and repair of the osteonecrotic lesion(s). Bone densitometry may provide a useful noninvasive measure of the therapeutic potential of these treatments. Dual energy x-ray absorptiometry (DEXA) is the gold standard for bone mass measurement. Although frequently used for assessment of osteoporosis and fracture risk, it has also been used to evaluate the extent of fracture healing.[45,46]

Bone grafting and cell-based therapies used as an adjunct to bone grafting pose a significant challenge to the use of DEXA to assess changes in bone density in the affected region. The density of the graft material (autograft, allograft, or a bone graft substitute such as tricalcium phosphate) may obscure the changes in osteogenesis within the defect.

Other potential sources of error in the use of DEXA include: the absorber (patient) thickness, the effect of bone distance from the imaging table, and the effect of fat content surrounding the bone.[46] While the application of DEXA to the study of lesion repair with osteonecrosis is reasonable, additional studies are needed to determine the sensitivity of this technique to small changes in lesion size over time.

New methodology

Imaging techniques continue to gain in sophistication. Gadolinium was first used as an enhancement agent to identify specific tissues in the 1980s. A few years later, it was applied to perfusion and tissue function. Gadolinium-enhanced MRI can be used to assess perfusion of the diseased tissue and its surrounding area.[47–50] Zerhouni and others studied its potential use in animal models to evaluate decreased blood flow to and from bone.[48,50] Although gadolinium-enhanced dynamic fast MRI has been adapted for use in humans,[47,49] it has not been used in clinical trials.

Doppler ultrasonography has also been used to estimate blood flow noninvasively. It has been adapted to the evaluation of bone[51–53] and has been applied to patients with Legg-Calve-Perthes disease[54,55] or osteonecrosis.[56,57] Lee and colleagues[57] found that the arterial pulsatility index and peak systolic velocity were significantly elevated in a patient cohort who had systemic lupus erythematosus, a group known to be at risk for osteonecrosis, when compared with healthy controls. Duchow and colleagues[56] used color Doppler imaging to evaluate the patency of the vessels of free vascularized grafts for the treatment of osteonecrosis; however, this report focused on the soft tissues and not the diseased bone.

Near infrared spectroscopy (NIRS) can be used to measure tissue oxygenation—an indirect measure of the circulation to the tissue under study. Khakha and colleagues[58] using NIRS to evaluate spinal injuries were able to detect a significant difference in several blood parameters during the hyperemic response to below-knee arterial occlusion. This technique has also been used to monitor the vascularity of vascularized free fibular grafts for mandibular reconstruction.[59] Further study is needed to determine whether it can successfully be adapted to osteonecrosis, particularly of the hip.[60]

Positron emission tomography (PET) is a nuclear medicine technique that combines tomographic imaging and real-time quantification of biologic processes depending on the type of radiolabeled marker used.[61,62] Schiepers and colleagues and Dasa and colleagues have used it to evaluate osteonecrosis of the hip. Using ^{18}F, Schiepers and colleagues[62] evaluated bone blood flow and the fluoride influx rate in five patients with osteonecrosis. They were able to measure bone blood flow as low as 0.02 mL/min/mL. They reported that a difference in the ratio of the abnormal to normal head of at least 2 for the bone blood flow or influx rate is needed to evaluate treatment. Dasa and colleagues[61] used PET to diagnose changes in the acetabulum that may not have been picked up using more traditional methodologies.

BIOMARKERS

Recent interest has centered on identifying biomarkers for the analysis of osteonecrosis; however, most of the studies have focused on biomarkers of cartilage degradation because obtaining synovial fluid from the affected joint is feasible.[63,64] Because changes in the cartilage are not observed until the later stages of osteonecrosis, this method is not likely to be useful for studies involving the treatment of early stages of the disease. Several potential biomarkers for bone turnover have been evaluated in other musculoskeletal diseases (**Box 2**). Berger and colleagues[65] have looked at biomarkers for SPONK (spontaneous osteonecrosis of the knee), which is a unique disease unlikely to be "true" osteonecrosis. Borgor and others[66] have also evaluated biomarkers in core biopsies taken from patients with bone marrow edema syndrome of the hip. They found elevated levels of several biomarkers of bone formation that were associated with increased bone turnover. Although bone marrow edema is commonly observed with osteonecrosis, bone marrow edema syndrome may be a distinctly different disease. In an evaluation of core biopsies from osteonecrosis patients, Radke and colleagues[67] found that VEGF and CYR61 were highly expressed in the edematous areas, whereas CTGF was noted in the areas with marrow fibrosis and edema. This investigation was a histologic study. Whether circulating levels of these markers will reflect the localized environment around the lesion remains to be investigated. Additional studies of levels of biomarkers of bone formation that are

specific to the different stages of osteonecrosis are needed before biomarkers will be a useful tool to study treatment of this disease.

SUMMARY

Although several tests can be used to evaluate the effect of a specific treatment for osteonecrosis, the definitive assessment will likely remain whether the disease progresses to the point that major surgery (eg, bone grafting including vascularized fibular grafting, resurfacing, and total joint arthroplasty) is required to relieve pain and restore function. A panel of assessment tools is warranted because the questions addressed by each differ, and more information will be gained by a more comprehensive approach. As we gain a better understanding of the pathogenesis of the disease, other more definitive outcome measures such as

---

Box 2
Potential biomarkers[107,108]

Bone formation

Alkaline phosphatase, total

Alkaline phosphatase, bone specific

Osteocalcin (OC)

C-terminal propeptide of type I procollagen (PICP)

N-terminal propeptide of type I procollagen (PINP)

Bone resorption

Hydroxyproline, total and dialyzable (Hyp)

Hydroxylysine-glycosides (HLG)

Pyridinoline, total (Pyr)

Pyridinoline, free (f-Pyr)

Deoxypyridinoline, total (dPyr)

Deoxypyridinoline, free (f-dPyr)

Carboxyterminal cross-linked telopeptide of type I collagen (ICTP, CTx-MMP)

Carboxyterminal cross-linked telopeptide of type I collagen (CTx-I)

Aminoterminal cross-linked telopeptide of type I collagen (NTx-I)

Collagen I alpha 1 helicoidal peptide (HELP)

Bone sialoprotein (BSP)

Osteocalcin fragments (ufOC, U-Mid-OC, U-LongOC)

Tartrate-resistant acid phosphatase (TRAP)

Cathepsins

biomarkers or imaging techniques may prove to be of utility in the study of various treatments for osteonecrosis.

REFERENCES

1. Stulberg B. Criteria for establishing the natural history of osteonecrosis of the femoral head. In: Urbaniak J, Jones JP, editors. Osteonecrosis—etiology, diagnosis, and treatment. Rosemont (IL): American Academy of Orthopaedic Surgeons; 1997. p. 59–65.
2. Bellamy N. Musculoskeletal clinical metrology. Boston: Kluwer Academic Publishers; 1993.
3. Harris WH. Traumatic arthritis of the hip after dislocation and acetabular fractures: treatment by mold arthroplasty. An end-result study using a new method of result evaluation. J Bone Joint Surg Am 1969;51(4):737–55.
4. Merle D'Aubigne R, Postel M. Functional results of hip arthroplasty with acrylic prosthesis. J Bone Joint Surg Am 1954;36A:451–76.
5. Bellamy N, Buchanan WW, Goldsmith CH, et al. Validation study of WOMAC: a health status instrument for measuring clinically important patient relevant outcomes to antirheumatic drug therapy in patients with osteoarthritis of the hip or knee. J Rheumatol 1988;15(12):1833–40.
6. Johanson NA, Liang MH, Daltroy L, et al. American Academy of Orthopaedic Surgeons lower limb outcomes assessment instruments: reliability, validity, and sensitivity to change. J Bone Joint Surg Am 2004;86-A(5):902–9.
7. Ware JE Jr, Sherbourne CD. The MOS 36-item short-form health survey (SF-36). I. Conceptual framework and item selection. Med Care 1992; 30(6):473–83.
8. Sayed-Noor AS, Englund E, Wretenberg P, et al. Pressure-pain threshold algometric measurement in patients with greater trochanteric pain after total hip arthroplasty. Clin J Pain 2008;24(3):232–6.
9. Kong J, Kaptchuk TJ, Polich G, et al. Placebo analgesia: findings from brain imaging studies and emerging hypotheses. Rev Neurosci 2007; 18(3–4):173–90.
10. Meenan RF, Pincus T. The status of patient status measures. J Rheumatol 1987;14(3):411–4.
11. Beaule PE, Dorey FJ, Hoke R, et al. The value of patient activity level in the outcome of total hip arthroplasty. J Arthroplasty 2006;21(4):547–52.
12. Hunsaker FG, Cioffi DA, Amadio PC, et al. The American Academy of Orthopaedic Surgeons outcomes instruments: normative values from the general population. J Bone Joint Surg Am 2002; 84-A(2):208–15.
13. Riddle DL, Stratford PW, Bowman DH. Findings of extensive variation in the types of outcome measures used in hip and knee replacement clinical trials: a systematic review. Arthritis Rheum 2008;59(6):876–83.
14. Pollard B, Johnston M, Dieppe P. What do osteoarthritis health outcome instruments measure? Impairment, activity limitation, or participation restriction? J Rheumatol 2006;33(4):757–63.
15. Ficat RP. Idiopathic bone necrosis of the femoral head: early diagnosis and treatment. J Bone Joint Surg Br 1985;67(1):3–9.
16. Ficat RP, Arlet J. In: Hungerford DS, editor. Ischemia and necrosis of bone. Baltimore: Williams and Wilkins; 1980.
17. Steinberg ME, Hayken GD, Steinberg DR. A quantitative system for staging avascular necrosis. J Bone Joint Surg Br 1995;77(1):34–41.
18. Steinberg ME, Steinberg DR. Classification systems for osteonecrosis: an overview. Orthop Clin North Am 2004;35(3):273–83.
19. Gardeniers J. ARCO Committee on Terminology and Staging. Report on the committee meeting at Santiago de Compostella. ARCO Newsletter 1993; 5:79–82.
20. Sugano N, Atsumi T, Ohzono K, et al. The 2001 revised criteria for diagnosis, classification, and staging of idiopathic osteonecrosis of the femoral head. J Orthop Sci 2002;7(5):601–5.
21. Berend KR, Gunneson EE, Urbaniak JR. Free vascularized fibular grafting for the treatment of postcollapse osteonecrosis of the femoral head. J Bone Joint Surg Am 2003;85-A(6):987–93.
22. Marcus ND, Enneking WF, Massam RA. The silent hip in idiopathic aseptic necrosis: treatment by bone-grafting. J Bone Joint Surg Am 1973;55(7): 1351–66.
23. Mont MA, Marulanda GA, Jones LC, et al. Systematic analysis of classification systems for osteonecrosis of the femoral head. J Bone Joint Surg Am 2006;88(Suppl 3):16–26.
24. Mont MA, Jones LC, Sotereanos DG, et al. Understanding and treating osteonecrosis of the femoral head. Instr Course Lect 2000;49:169–85.
25. Plakseychuk AY, Shah M, Varitimidis SE, et al. Classification of osteonecrosis of the femoral head: reliability, reproducibility, and prognostic value. Clin Orthop Relat Res 2001;386:34–41.
26. Schmitt-Sody M, Kirchhoff C, Mayer W, et al. Avascular necrosis of the femoral head: inter- and intraobserver variations of Ficat and ARCO classifications. Int Orthop 2008;32(3):283–7.
27. Smith SW, Meyer RA, Connor PM, et al. Interobserver reliability and intraobserver reproducibility of the modified Ficat classification system of osteonecrosis of the femoral head. J Bone Joint Surg Am 1996;78(11):1702–6.
28. Stevens K, Tao C, Lee SU, et al. Subchondral fractures in osteonecrosis of the femoral

head: comparison of radiography, CT, and MR imaging. AJR Am J Roentgenol 2003;180(2):363–8.

29. Dorey F, Amstutz HC. Survivorship analysis in the evaluation of joint replacement. J Arthroplasty 1986;1(1):63–9.

30. Koo KH, Kim R, Kim YS, et al. Risk period for developing osteonecrosis of the femoral head in patients on steroid treatment. Clin Rheumatol 2002;21(4): 299–303.

31. Suk M, Norvell DC, Hanson B, et al. Evidence-based orthopaedic surgery: what is evidence without the outcomes? J Am Acad Orthop Surg 2008; 16(3):123–9.

32. Soderman P, Malchau H. Is the Harris hip score system useful to study the outcome of total hip replacement? Clin Orthop Relat Res 2001;384: 189–97.

33. Swiontkowski MF, Engelberg R, Martin DP, et al. Short musculoskeletal function assessment questionnaire: validity, reliability, and responsiveness. J Bone Joint Surg Am 1999;81(9):1245–60.

34. Bryant MJ, Kernohan WG, Nixon JR, et al. A statistical analysis of hip scores. J Bone Joint Surg Br 1993;75(5):705–9.

35. Dougados M. Monitoring osteoarthritis progression and therapy. Osteoarthritis Cartilage 2004; 12(Suppl A):S55–60.

36. Cherian SF, Laorr A, Saleh KJ, et al. Quantifying the extent of femoral head involvement in osteonecrosis. J Bone Joint Surg Am 2003;85-A(2): 309–15.

37. Mont MA, Jones LC, Pacheco I, et al. Radiographic predictors of outcome of core decompression for hips with osteonecrosis stage III. Clin Orthop Relat Res 1998;354:159–68.

38. Nishii T, Sugano N, Ohzono K, et al. Significance of lesion size and location in the prediction of collapse of osteonecrosis of the femoral head: a new three-dimensional quantification using magnetic resonance imaging. J Orthop Res 2002;20(1): 130–6.

39. Steinberg ME, Bands RE, Parry S, et al. Does lesion size affect the outcome in avascular necrosis? Clin Orthop Relat Res 1999;367:262–71.

40. Hernigou P, Lambotte JC. Volumetric analysis of osteonecrosis of the femur. Anatomical correlation using MRI. J Bone Joint Surg Br 2001;83(5): 672–5.

41. Kishida Y, Nishii T, Sugano N, et al. Measurement of lesion area and volume by three-dimensional spoiled gradient-echo MR imaging in osteonecrosis of the femoral head. J Orthop Res 2003;21(5): 850–8.

42. Steinberg DR, Steinberg ME, Garino JP, et al. Determining lesion size in osteonecrosis of the femoral head. J Bone Joint Surg Am 2006;88(Suppl 3): 27–34.

43. Koo KH, Kim R. Quantifying the extent of osteonecrosis of the femoral head: a new method using MRI. J Bone Joint Surg Br 1995;77(6):875–80.

44. Takao M, Sugano N, Nishii T, et al. Longitudinal quantitative evaluation of lesion size change in femoral head osteonecrosis using three-dimensional magnetic resonance imaging and image registration. J Orthop Res 2006;24(6):1231–9.

45. Iida Y, Kuroda T, Kitano T, et al. Dexa-measured bone density changes over time after intertrochanteric hip fractures. The Kobe Journal of Medical Sciences 2000;46:1–12.

46. Markel MD, Chao EY. Noninvasive monitoring techniques for quantitative description of callus mineral content and mechanical properties. Clinical Orthopaedics and Related Research 1993; 293:37–45.

47. Bluemke DA, Petri M, Zerhouni EA. Femoral head perfusion and composition: MR imaging and spectroscopic evaluation of patients with systemic lupus erythematosus and at risk for avascular necrosis. Radiology 1995;197(2):433–8.

48. Cova M, Kang YS, Tsukamoto H, et al. Bone marrow perfusion evaluated with gadolinium-enhanced dynamic fast MR imaging in a dog model. Radiology 1991;179(2):535–9.

49. Schedel H, Schneller A, Vogl T, et al. [Dynamic magnetic resonance tomography (MRI): a follow-up study after femur core decompression and instillation of recombinant human bone morphogenetic protein-2 (rhBMP-2) in avascular femur head necrosis]. Rontgenpraxis 2000;53(1):16–24 [in German].

50. Tsukamoto H, Kang YS, Jones LC, et al. Evaluation of marrow perfusion in the femoral head by dynamic magnetic resonance imaging: effect of venous occlusion in a dog model. Invest Radiol 1992;27(4):275–81.

51. Espahbodi S, Humphries K, Dore C, et al. Colour Doppler ultrasound in the assessment of lumbar spine blood flow in patients with low back pain. In: ARCO International Meeting on Bone Circulation. London, September 15–17, 2005.

52. Graif M, Schweitzer ME, Nazarian L, et al. Color Doppler hemodynamic evaluation of flow to normal hip. J Ultrasound Med 1998;17(5):275–80 [quiz, 281–2].

53. Keast-Butler O, Shenava Y, Rajaratnam S, et al. In vivo measurement of tibial blood flow during distraction osteogenesis using Doppler ultrasonography. In: ARCO International Meeting on Bone Circulation. London, 2005.

54. Doria AS, Cunha FG, Modena M, et al. Legg-Calve-Perthes disease: multipositional power Doppler sonography of the proximal femoral vascularity. Pediatr Radiol 2008;38(4):392–402.

55. Doria AS, Guarniero R, Molnar LJ, et al. Three-dimensional (3D) contrast-enhanced power Doppler

imaging in Legg-Calve-Perthes disease. Pediatr Radiol 2000;30(12):871–4.

56. Duchow J, Kubale R, Hopf T. Color Doppler imaging assessment of blood flow in vascularized pedicle grafts for avascular necrosis of the femoral head: angiographic correlation. J Ultrasound Med 1998;17(8):509–12.

57. Lee CW, Kim HJ, Shin MJ. Evaluation of haemodynamic flow to the hip in patients with systemic lupus erythematosus. Scand J Rheumatol 2007;36(1):36–9.

58. Khakha R, Bloomer Z, Bain D, et al. Differences in the reactive hyperaemia response of bone in able-bodied and spinal injured persons using near infrared spectroscopy. In: ARCO International Symposium on the Circulation of Bone. London, September 15–17, 2005.

59. Cai ZG, Zhang J, Zhang JG, et al. Evaluation of near infrared spectroscopy in monitoring postoperative regional tissue oxygen saturation for fibular flaps. J Plast Reconstr Aesthet Surg 2008;61(3):289–96.

60. McCarthy I. The physiology of bone blood flow: a review. J Bone Joint Surg Am 2006;88(Suppl 3):4–9.

61. Dasa V, Adbel-Nabi H, Anders MJ, et al. F-18 fluoride positron emission tomography of the hip for osteonecrosis. Clin Orthop Relat Res 2008;466(5):1081–6.

62. Schiepers C, Broos P, Miserez M, et al. Measurement of skeletal flow with positron emission tomography and 18F-fluoride in femoral head osteonecrosis. Arch Orthop Trauma Surg 1998;118(3):131–5.

63. Jingushi S, Lohmander LS, Shinmei M, et al. Markers of joint tissue turnover in joint fluids from hips with osteonecrosis of the femoral head. J Orthop Res 2000;18(5):728–33.

64. Kato S, Yamada H, Terada N, et al. Joint biomarkers in idiopathic femoral head osteonecrosis: comparison with hip osteoarthritis. J Rheumatol 2005;32(8):1518–23.

65. Berger CE, Kroner A, Kristen KH, et al. Spontaneous osteonecrosis of the knee: biochemical markers of bone turnover and pathohistology. Osteoarthritis Cartilage 2005;13(8):716–21.

66. Berger CE, Kroner AH, Minai-Pour MB, et al. Biochemical markers of bone metabolism in bone marrow edema syndrome of the hip. Bone 2003;33(3):346–51.

67. Radke S, Battmann A, Jatzke S, et al. Expression of the angiomatrix and angiogenic proteins CYR61, CTGF, and VEGF in osteonecrosis of the femoral head. J Orthop Res 2006;24(5):945–52.

68. Brooks R. EuroQol: the current state of play. Health Policy 1996;37(1):53–72.

69. Hunt SM, McKenna SP, McEwen J, et al. The Nottingham Health Profile: subjective health status and medical consultations. Soc Sci Med [A] 1981;15(3 Pt 1):221–9.

70. Thomee R, Grimby G, Wright BD, et al. Rasch analysis of Visual Analog Scale measurements before and after treatment of patellofemoral pain syndrome in women. Scand J Rehabil Med 1995;27(3):145–51.

71. Meenan RF, Gertman PM, Mason JH. Measuring health status in arthritis: the arthritis impact measurement scales. Arthritis Rheum 1980;23(2):146–52.

72. Fries JF, Spitz P, Kraines RG, et al. Measurement of patient outcome in arthritis. Arthritis Rheum 1980;23(2):137–45.

73. Lequesne MG, Mery C, Samson M, et al. Indexes of severity for osteoarthritis of the hip and knee. Validation–value in comparison with other assessment tests. Scand J Rheumatol Suppl 1987;65:85–9.

74. Tugwell P, Bombardier C, Buchanan WW, et al. The MACTAR Patient Preference Disability Questionnaire–an individualized functional priority approach for assessing improvement in physical disability in clinical trials in rheumatoid arthritis. J Rheumatol 1987;14(3):446–51.

75. Dawson J, Fitzpatrick R, Carr A, et al. Questionnaire on the perceptions of patients about total hip replacement. J Bone Joint Surg Br 1996;78(2):185–90.

76. Zahiri CA, Schmalzried TP, Szuszczewicz ES, et al. Assessing activity in joint replacement patients. J Arthroplasty 1998;13(8):890–5.

77. Stulberg BN, Davis AW, Bauer TW, et al. Osteonecrosis of the femoral head: a prospective randomized treatment protocol. Clin Orthop Relat Res 1991;268:140–51.

78. Fairbank AC, Bhatia D, Jinnah RH, et al. Long-term results of core decompression for ischaemic necrosis of the femoral head. J Bone Joint Surg Br 1995;77(1):42–9.

79. Koo KH, Kim R, Ko GH, et al. Preventing collapse in early osteonecrosis of the femoral head: a randomised clinical trial of core decompression. J Bone Joint Surg Br 1995;77(6):870–4.

80. Kane SM, Ward WA, Jordan LC, et al. Vascularized fibular grafting compared with core decompression in the treatment of femoral head osteonecrosis. Orthopedics 1996;19(10):869–72.

81. Chang MC, Chen TH, Lo WH. Core decompression in treating ischemic necrosis of the femoral head. Zhonghua Yi Xue Za Zhi (Taipei) 1997;60(3):130–6.

82. Mazieres B, Marin F, Chiron P, et al. Influence of the volume of osteonecrosis on the outcome of core decompression of the femoral head. Ann Rheum Dis 1997;56(12):747–50.

83. Mont MA, Fairbank AC, Petri M, et al. Core decompression for osteonecrosis of the femoral head in systemic lupus erythematosus. Clin Orthop Relat Res 1997;334:91–7.

84. Powell ET, Lanzer WL, Mankey MG. Core decompression for early osteonecrosis of the hip in high risk patients. Clin Orthop Relat Res 1997;335:181–9 [in French].

85. Iorio R, Healy WL, Abramowitz AJ, et al. Clinical outcome and survivorship analysis of core decompression for early osteonecrosis of the femoral head. J Arthroplasty 1998;13(1):34–41.

86. Scully SP, Aaron RK, Urbaniak JR. Survival analysis of hips treated with core decompression or vascularized fibular grafting because of avascular necrosis. J Bone Joint Surg Am 1998;80(9):1270–5.

87. Wirtz C, Zilkens KW, Adam G, et al. [MRI-controlled outcome after core decompression of the femur head in aseptic osteonecrosis and transient bone marrow edema]. Z Orthop Ihre Grenzgeb 1998;136(2):138–46 [in German].

88. Bozic KJ, Zurakowski D, Thornhill TS. Survivorship analysis of hips treated with core decompression for nontraumatic osteonecrosis of the femoral head. J Bone Joint Surg Am 1999;81(2):200–9.

89. Chen CH, Chang JK, Huang KY, et al. Core decompression for osteonecrosis of the femoral head at pre-collapse stage. Kaohsiung J Med Sci 2000;16(2):76–82.

90. Maniwa S, Nishikori T, Furukawa S, et al. Evaluation of core decompression for early osteonecrosis of the femoral head. Arch Orthop Trauma Surg 2000;120(5–6):241–4.

91. Specchiulli F. Core decompression in the treatment of necrosis of the femoral head: long-term results. Chir Organi Mov 2000;85(4):395–402.

92. Yoon TR, Song EK, Rowe SM, et al. Failure after core decompression in osteonecrosis of the femoral head. Int Orthop 2001;24(6):316–8.

93. Aigner N, Schneider W, Eberl V, et al. Core decompression in early stages of femoral head osteonecrosis–an MRI-controlled study. Int Orthop 2002;26(1):31–5.

94. Hernigou P, Beaujean F. Treatment of osteonecrosis with autologous bone marrow grafting. Clin Orthop Relat Res 2002;405:14–23.

95. Gangji V, Hauzeur JP, Matos C, et al. Treatment of osteonecrosis of the femoral head with implantation of autologous bone-marrow cells: a pilot study. J Bone Joint Surg Am 2004;86-A(6):1153–60.

96. Lieberman JR, Conduah A, Urist MR. Treatment of osteonecrosis of the femoral head with core decompression and human bone morphogenetic protein. Clin Orthop Relat Res 2004;429:139–45.

97. Agarwala S, Jain D, Joshi VR, et al. Efficacy of alendronate, a bisphosphonate, in the treatment of AVN of the hip: a prospective open-label study. Rheumatology (Oxford) 2005;44(3):352–9.

98. Bellot F, Havet E, Gabrion A, et al. [Core decompression of the femoral head for avascular necrosis]. Rev Chir Orthop Reparatrice Appar Mot 2005;91(2):114–23 [in French].

99. Lai KA, Shen WJ, Yang CY, et al. The use of alendronate to prevent early collapse of the femoral head in patients with nontraumatic osteonecrosis: a randomized clinical study. J Bone Joint Surg Am 2005;87(10):2155–9.

100. Tsao AK, Roberson JR, Christie MJ, et al. Biomechanical and clinical evaluations of a porous tantalum implant for the treatment of early stage osteonecrosis. J Bone Joint Surg Am 2005;87(Suppl 2):22–7.

101. Ha YC, Jung WH, Kim JR, et al. Prediction of collapse in femoral head osteonecrosis: a modified Kerboul method with use of magnetic resonance images. J Bone Joint Surg Am 2006;88(Suppl 3):35–40.

102. Neumayr LD, Aquilar C, Earles AN, et al. Physical therapy alone compared with core decompression and physical therapy for femoral head osteonecrosis in sickle cell disease: results of a multicenter study at a mean of three years after treatment. J Bone Joint Surg Am 2006;88(12):2573–82.

103. Nishii T, Sugano N, Miki H, et al. Does alendronate prevent collapse in osteonecrosis of the femoral head? Clin Orthop Relat Res 2006;443:273–9.

104. Veillette CJ, Mehdian H, Schemitsch EH, et al. Survivorship analysis and radiographic outcome following tantalum rod insertion for osteonecrosis of the femoral head. J Bone Joint Surg Am 2006;88(Suppl 3):48–55.

105. Shuler MS, Rooks MD, Roberson JR. Porous tantalum implant in early osteonecrosis of the hip: preliminary report on operative, survival, and outcomes results. J Arthroplasty 2007;22(1):26–31.

106. Song WS, Yoo JJ, Kim YM, et al. Results of multiple drilling compared with those of conventional methods of core decompression. Clin Orthop Relat Res 2007;454:139–46.

107. Looker AC, Bauer DC, Chesnut CH 3rd, et al. Clinical use of biochemical markers of bone remodeling: current status and future directions. Osteoporos Int 2000;11(6):467–80.

108. Seibel MJ. Clinical application of biochemical markers of bone turnover. Arq Bras Endocrinol Metabol 2006;50(4):603–20.

Osteonecrosis of the Knee: A Review of Three Disorders

Michael G. Zywiel, MD[a], Mike S. McGrath, MD[a],
Thorsten M. Seyler, MD[b], David R. Marker, BS[a],
Peter M. Bonutti, MD[c], Michael A. Mont, MD[a],*

KEYWORDS

- Osteonecrosis • Avascular necrosis • Core decompression
- Osteochondral autograft transfer • Knee pain
- Spontaneous osteonecrosis of the knee • Knee arthroscopy

Osteonecrosis (ON) of the knee is a debilitating disease that is poorly understood. Originally described as a single disorder, it encompasses three distinct conditions: spontaneous osteonecrosis of the knee (SPONK), secondary ON of the knee, and postarthroscopic ON of the knee. This article reviews the current knowledge of these distinct conditions by describing their etiology, pathology, and pathogenesis in addition to their clinical and radiographic presentations. The various treatment options available for each condition are reviewed, with a discussion of their rationale and indications and a summary of results with various techniques. A thorough understanding of these conditions and their distinguishing features is critical to selecting the best treatment option for an individual patient.

ON of the knee was first described by Ahlbäck and colleagues[1] in 1968. Our present understanding of the disease encompasses a few distinct conditions: SPONK, which typically affects a single condyle in older patients; true ON, which is most commonly seen in younger patients after exposure to corticosteroids and presents with several simultaneous foci in the distal femur or proximal tibia; and postarthroscopic ON, which presents in a condyle after arthroscopic surgery. In addition, true ON can occur after trauma, radiation, or other rare disorders. Although different gender and location biases have been reported for these conditions, all three can affect women or men and can involve the distal femora, proximal tibiae, or both.

Because of the low incidence of these conditions, there are few reports on series of 50 or more cases and there are no prospective studies comparing the efficacy of different treatment methods. Nevertheless, considerable progress has been made in understanding the underlying origins of these disorders and in examining the outcomes of various surgical and nonsurgical treatments. The present work serves as a review of the current knowledge to assist clinicians in the management of these conditions.

It is often difficult to distinguish between these disorders because they can present with seemingly nonspecific knee pain and equivocal findings on physical and radiologic examination. However, the authors believe they should not be confused because they can be clearly demarcated. Whereas SPONK presents as unilateral disease in older patients with a single focus and no associated factors, secondary ON presents as bilateral disease in younger patients with multiple joint involvement and associated diseases or factors. ON after arthroscopy affects one or both femoral condyles in the operated knee. **Table 1** outlines a comparison between SPONK, secondary ON, and postarthroscopic ON. These conditions differ in their

[a] Center for Joint Preservation and Reconstruction, Rubin Institute for Advanced Orthopedics, Sinai Hospital of Baltimore, 2401 West Belvedere Avenue, Baltimore, MD 21215, USA
[b] Department of Orthopaedic Surgery, Wake Forest University School of Medicine, Medical Center Boulevard, Winston-Salem, NC 27157, USA
[c] Bonutti Clinic, 1303 West Evergreen Avenue, Effingham, IL 62401, USA
* Corresponding author.
E-mail address: mmont@lifebridgehealth.org (M.A. Mont).

Orthop Clin N Am 40 (2009) 193–211
doi:10.1016/j.ocl.2008.10.010

Table 1
Comparison of spontaneous osteonecrosis, secondary osteonecrosis, and postarthroscopic osteonecrosis of the knee

Characteristic	Spontaneous Osteonecrosis of the Knee	Secondary Osteonecrosis of the Knee	Postarthroscopic Osteonecrosis	
Age (years)	55 and older	Younger than 45	No bias	
Gender	3:1 ♀:♂	♀ > ♂ with SLE as associated factor ♂ > ♀ with alcohol as associated factor	No bias	
Onset of pain	Sudden	Gradual	Sudden	
Bilaterality	<5%	>80%	Never	
No. lesions	One	Multiple	One	
Location on bone	Epiphysis	Epiphysis, metaphysis, and diaphysis	Epiphysis	
Condylar involvement	One condyle (femur 90%, tibia 10%)	Multiple condyles (femur 90%, tibia 20%)	One condyle (femur 95%)	
Femur and tibia affected	No	~20%	Never	
Other joint involvement	No	>90% (hip, shoulder, ankle)	No	
Associated factors	None	Corticosteroids, alcohol, tobacco, other	Arthroscopic surgery	
Associated diseases	None	SLE, sickle cell, caisson disease, Gaucher's disease, thrombophilia, hypofibrinolysis	None	
Pathologic findings	Fibrotic bone, healing fracture	Necrotic bone	After laser-assisted chondroplasty	Necrotic bone
			After mechanical debridement or meniscectomy	Fibrotic bone and healing fracture

Abbreviations: SLE, systemic lupus erythematosus; ♀, women; ♂, men.

etiology, diagnosis, and treatment, and it is important to recognize these differences to be able to manage the disease most appropriately and achieve the best possible patient outcomes. The following review addresses each disorder separately.

SPONTANEOUS OSTEONECROSIS OF THE KNEE
Etiology, Pathology, and Pathogenesis

SPONK is a disorder of unknown etiology. Some researchers believe that there is an underlying traumatic cause, with the primary insult eventually leading to collapse of the affected region. Several reports have demonstrated the presence of subchondral fractures in an affected condyle,[2–4] with a recent report suggesting that this precedes the development of necrotic tissue.[5] Some researchers have postulated that after the traumatic event, fluid enters the intracondylar region of the bone through the fracture gap, leading to increased intraosseous pressure, decreased blood perfusion, and eventual focal osseous ischemia.[6,7] However, other investigators report no necrotic tissue in the affected region. Yamamoto and Bullough[2] reported histopathologic results in a group of 14 patients with SPONK, in which 3 patients had a subchondral fracture with no evidence of necrosis, 6 patients had a subchondral fracture with focal necrosis distal to the fracture line only, and 5 patients had indeterminate findings attributable to detachment of the affected fragment. They concluded that necrosis was not the primary condition but only secondary to a subchondral insufficiency fracture. Mears and colleagues[8] reported no necrotic bone in the affected region on examination of histopathologic samples from 23 of 24 patients diagnosed with SPONK but did find osteoarthritis in 18 patients (75%) and osteoporosis in 18 patients (75%). These reports imply that the rarely identifiable bone death found is attributable to physiologic bone resorption and remodeling that takes place after a bone fracture and is not true ON, which is then a misnomer.

No medical, genetic, or pharmacologic factors have been identified to be associated with SPONK. In the authors' experience, less than 10% of patients report any history of trauma to the affected knee. However, given the demographics of the affected patients and the high incidence of insufficiency fractures among older persons, especially postmenopausal women,[9] it is understandable why many patients cannot identify a precipitating event or associate the onset of knee pain with an unrelated event.

Diagnostic Methods

SPONK has been classically described as being localized to the medial femoral condyle. However, the lateral femoral condyle and tibial condyles, as well as the patella, are also susceptible.[10–12] Patients presenting with a clinical suspicion of SPONK are typically older (>55 years of age), with women outnumbering men 3 to 1. Patients usually report the sudden onset of severe unilateral knee pain localized to the affected condyle, with the pain usually reported to be worse at night or with weight bearing. An effusion may be present, and range of motion may be somewhat limited secondary to the pain or effusion. Unless there are any preexisting problems, the results of examination of the knee for instability are normal.

Radiographic changes vary dramatically depending on the stage and severity of the disease. Lucencies in the epiphyseal region are typical findings on anteroposterior (AP) and lateral radiographs of the knee. However, the x-ray appearance ranges from completely normal in early stages of the disease to collapse of the affected condyle with degenerative changes of the opposite articular surface in the most advanced stages.

Magnetic resonance imaging (MRI) is extremely sensitive and specific in detecting SPONK, with low signal in the affected area on T1-weighted images and a high signal margin of the affected area on T2-weighted images.[13] These changes can be evident in the early stages of the disease before any abnormalities are visible on plain radiographs.

Several reports have suggested that radionucleotide scintimetry is effective in the detection of early-stage SPONK, with increased update visible on scans before the appearance of visible changes on plain radiographs.[14–16] However, other reports found a low sensitivity of these scans for secondary ON,[17] suggesting that they may also have limited benefit in diagnosing SPONK. Regardless, it is not clear whether this information aids in treating the patient. Clinical symptoms suggestive of SPONK should be treated with protected weight bearing and analgesia regardless of the outcome of scintimetry, with further treatment indicated only for stages of SPONK defined by visible changes on radiographs.

Koshino[18] developed the first staging system, as shown in **Table 2**, based on a combination of clinical and radiographic indications. The authors prefer to stage using the Ficat and Arlet radiographic system for the hip as adapted for the knee, which is also shown in **Table 2**.[19–21] There are four stages of disease progression defined in the Ficat and Arlet system. Each stage is determined by a combination of three criteria: the level of joint space narrowing, evidence of condyle contour collapse, and trabecular pattern (**Figs. 1–4**).

The size of the lesion has been described as a prognostic factor in SPONK. Lesions can be sized using one of three methods originally developed for secondary ON. Motohashi and colleagues[22] measured the greatest width of the lesion in millimeters on the AP and lateral radiographs, a system first described by Ahlbäck and colleagues.[1] Lesions measuring less than 10 mm were described as small, and those measuring more than 10 mm were described as large. Aglietti and colleagues[23] estimated the size of the lesion by measuring the greatest width of the lesion on the AP and lateral radiographs, as shown in **Fig. 5**, in addition to measuring the width of the lesion on the AP radiograph as a ratio of the total width of the affected condyle. Their study considered lucencies with an area greater than 5 cm^2 or a size ratio greater than 0.40 as large lesions, which had a poor prognosis. Kerboul and colleagues[24] outlined lesions of the hip on AP and lateral radiographs and then measured the angle of the arc tangential to the two sides of the lesion and with the fulcrum at the physeal scar on each projection. This size measurement for the hip

Table 2
Comparison of Koshino and modified Ficat and Arlet staging systems for the knee

Stage	Koshino			Modified Ficat and Arlet		
	Radiographic Changes	Appearance on Direct Visualization	Clinical Presentation	Joint Space	Condyle Contour	Trabecular Pattern
I	Normal radiograph	Not specified	Patient complains of knee pain	Normal	Normal	Mottled areas of osteoporosis
II	Radiolucency in subchondral weight-bearing area, with cortical sclerosis distal to lucency	Normal or flattened articular cartilage, with or without shallow fissures	Not specified	Normal	Normal	Wedge sclerosis
III	Expanded lucency surrounded by sclerotic halo, calcified collapsed subchondral bone plate	Cartilage flap attached to necrotic lesion, with or without cartilaginous free bodies	Not specified	Normal or slightly decreased	Subchondral collapse	Sequestrum appearance
IV	Osteophytes and osteosclerosis on affected condyle and ipsilateral tibial plateau	Not specified	Not specified	Decreased	Collapse	Extensive destruction

Data from Refs.[18–21]

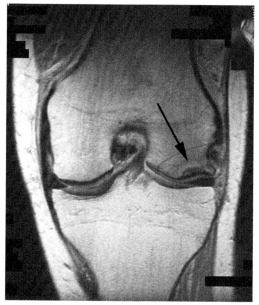

Fig. 1. Stage 1 SPONK lesion of the lateral femoral condyle (*arrow*) seen on T1-weighted MRI, with a high-signal margin surrounding the low-signal lesion.

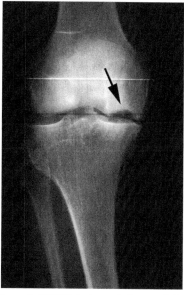

Fig. 3. Stage 3 SPONK lesion of the medial femoral condyle (*arrow*), with subchondral collapse and decreased joint space.

was modified to apply to the knee by Mont and colleagues[25] in a similar manner by summing the angles in both views, as shown in **Fig. 6**. The two angles were added to calculate the combined necrotic angle. They classified lesions of 150° or less as small, of 151° to 249° as intermediate, and of 250° or greater as large, with the best prognosis reserved for small early-stage lesions.

Treatment of Spontaneous Osteonecrosis of the Knee

There are various treatment methods for SPONK, based on staging and lesion size, ranging from nonoperative treatment and joint-preserving methods to unicompartmental and total knee arthroplasty (TKA). **Fig. 7** illustrates the treatment

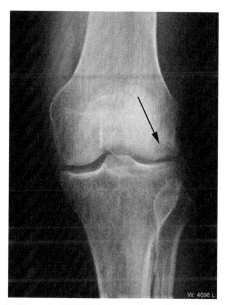

Fig. 2. Stage 2 SPONK lesion of the lateral femoral condyle (*arrow*), with visible epiphyseal lucency but no subchondral collapse.

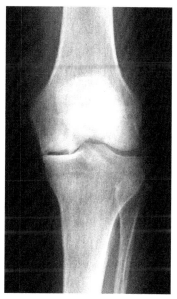

Fig. 4. Stage 4 SPONK lesion of the medial femoral condyle, with condylar collapse and joint space destruction.

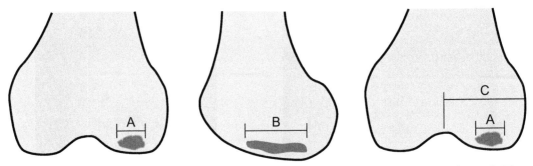

Fig. 5. Lesion size can be estimated by measuring the greatest width of the lucency on an AP radiograph (A) and multiplying it by the greatest length of the lucency on a lateral radiograph (B), in addition to the ratio of lesion width to total width of the affected condyle (A divided by C). (*Data from* Aglietti P, Insall JN, Buzzi R, et al. Idiopathic osteonecrosis of the knee. Aetiology, prognosis and treatment. J Bone Joint Surg Br 1983;65:589.)

algorithm favored by the authors, encompassing the individual treatment methods described in this section.

Nonoperative treatment

Initial treatment in precollapse disease is nonoperative, consisting of protected weight bearing and nonsteroidal anti-inflammatory drugs for analgesia as required, if tolerated. Uchio and colleagues[26] reported success with the use of a wedge insole to reduce weight bearing on the affected condyle. They followed 18 knees for a mean of 52 months (range: 36–183 months) and found initial and final mean Hospital for Special Surgery knee scores of 58.6 and 69.9, respectively, and mean radiologic reductions of necrotic area from 2.3 to 1.3 cm². The best results were achieved in small stage I and II lesions, with all 9 knees initially classified in those stages remaining at the same stage at final follow-up. Lotke and colleagues[27] reported that

32 (88.9%) of 36 knees with stage I SPONK and a mean follow-up of 3.5 years (range: 1–17 years) became and remained clinically asymptomatic over a range from 9 to 15 months after initial presentation after treatment with protected weight bearing and analgesia. Yates and colleagues[28] reported a mean time to recovery from clinical symptoms of knee pain of 4.8 months (range: 3–8 months) in all 20 knees with stage I SPONK treated with protected weight bearing or activity restriction and analgesia. Lesions resolved at a mean time of 8 months (range: 3–18 months) in all 19 patients for whom follow-up MRI scans were available, although the exact follow-up period was not reported.

In general, the results of multiple studies have suggested that most small lesions resolve with nonoperative treatment, medium-sized lesions may or may not resolve, and most large lesions collapse. Based on these results, nonoperative treatment should be attempted in patients

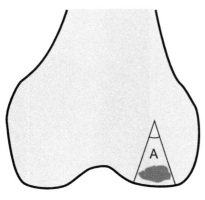
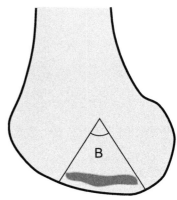

Fig. 6. Lesion size can also be estimated by measuring the angle of the arc tangential to both sides of the lesion in the AP radiograph (A) and summing it with the angle of the arc tangential to both sides of the lesion in the lateral radiograph (B). (*Adapted from* Mont MA, Baumgarten KM, Rifai A, et al. Atraumatic osteonecrosis of the knee. J Bone Joint Surg Am 2000;82:1282; with permission.)

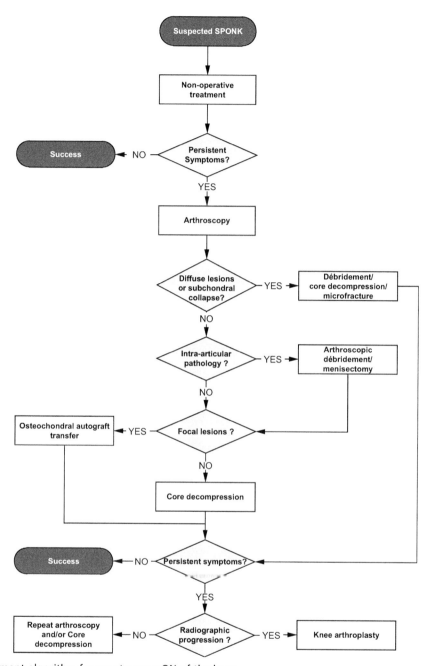

Fig. 7. Treatment algorithm for spontaneous ON of the knee.

diagnosed with SPONK with small and medium-sized lesions, with excellent results to be expected in patients presenting with early-stage small lesions.

Arthroscopy (with or without microfracture treatment)

Arthroscopic exploration of the knee allows the surgeon to visualize the lesions directly and to assess any other coexisting problems, such as meniscal tears. This allows for decision making regarding appropriate further treatment. This procedure is indicated in cases in which there is some question regarding the size or status of the cartilage defects in patients with more advanced disease or in which there is concern about other concomitant knee problems. Débridement or microfracture treatment of lesions can be performed during exploration if deemed appropriate, and core decompression or osteochondral autografting can be performed if indicated based on the arthroscopic findings.

Microfracture treatment involves intra-articular drilling of multiple small-diameter holes through the cartilage defect into the bone marrow under arthroscopic control. The rationale of this procedure is to stimulate the bone marrow to bring blood into the area of the cartilage defect and promote healing.[29] Akgun and colleagues[30] performed arthroscopic microfracture treatment, with concurrent partial meniscectomy in patients with meniscal tears, in 26 patients. At a mean follow-up of 27 months (range: 12–78 months), 96% of patients reported feeling better or much better on a four-point subjective patient response scale. However, 20 of the 26 patients remained at the same or worse radiographic stage, using the scale developed by Koshino (**Table 2**).[18] The authors have performed arthroscopic exploration with débridement and microfracture treatment in a few patients with articular cartilage defects but prefer to use osteochondral autologous transfer (OATS) techniques for treatment of chondral lesions when they are of an appropriate size (<20–30 mm in size).[31,32]

Osteochondral defect repair

Patients who fail to improve with conservative treatment or present with or progress to stage III or IV disease may benefit from surgical chondral defect repair. In this method, articular cartilage with subchondral bone is harvested from less weight-bearing surfaces and transplanted to the diseased areas. With this procedure, patients are treated with transplantation of autologous tissue in an attempt to preserve the native joint and avoid prosthetic implantation. This is indicated in patients with a localized and well-defined lesion, in which enough autologous osteochondral tissue can be harvested from noninvolved less weight-bearing articular surfaces to ensure coverage of the affected area. Several surgical repair systems have been anecdotally described, but the authors are not aware of any studies that have specifically assessed or compared these procedures for SPONK. The authors prefer to use an OATS procedure utilizing cylindric osteochondral grafts, as described by Hangody and colleagues[33] and shown in **Fig. 8**, with rehabilitation consisting of 4 weeks of partial weight bearing after surgery and progression to full weight bearing as tolerated. Overall, medium- to long-term results for repairing defects of the weight-bearing surfaces of the knee have been favorable, with Hangody and colleagues[34] reporting good to excellent clinical results in 92%

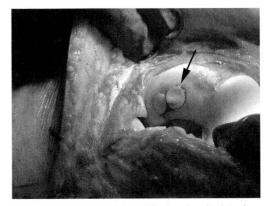

Fig. 8. Focal cartilage defect filled with cylindric chondral autografts (*arrow*) harvested from less weight-bearing areas of the femoral articular surface.

of 789 patients with femoral condylar implants and in 87% of 32 patients with tibial plateau implants. Clinical results were measured with modified Hospital for Special Surgery, modified Cincinnati, Lysholm, and International Cartilage Repair Society scores. Follow-up intervals were not specified in this report, but patients were operated on between February 1992 and August 2006, with the report published in April 2008. The authors have experienced similarly positive results for a carefully selected group of approximately 10 patients (N.G. Duany, M.G. Zywiel, M.S. McGrath, et al, unpublished data, 2008).

Core decompression

Core decompression involves surgical drilling of the affected femoral condyle using an extra-articular approach. This procedure relieves the elevated intraosseous pressure believed to contribute to ischemia in ON, and perhaps creates a vascular channel, facilitating physiologic healing of the lesion. It may be more appropriate for patients who have true or secondary ON. This procedure can be performed on an outpatient basis with percutaneous drilling. Fluoroscopic or arthroscopic guidance should be used to ensure good penetration of the drill into the affected epiphyseal region, avoiding any breach of the articular surface. Patients are kept at 50% weight bearing for 4 to 5 weeks and are then allowed full weight bearing with no high-impact activity until 1 year after surgery. As stated previously, this procedure is performed sometimes after diagnostic or therapeutic arthroscopy.

Forst and colleagues[35] reported on 16 patients treated with core decompression for early-stage SPONK. They found normalization of bone marrow signal and resolution of pain in 15 (94%) of 16 patients when followed for a mean of 35.4 months (range: 3–60 months). The authors are not aware of any other reports regarding treatment of SPONK with core decompression alone; however, in their own practice, they have found this procedure to be effective for early-stage disease before the appearance of chondral collapse (N.G. Duany, M.G. Zywiel, M.S. McGrath, et al, unpublished data, 2008).

High tibial osteotomy

The excellent outcomes reported with the newer generation unicompartmental implants have largely supplanted high tibial osteotomy (HTO) as a treatment modality for SPONK. However, it may still be a desirable mode of treatment in certain patients, especially those who would prefer to delay or avoid prosthetic implantation because of a combination of relatively young age and high activity levels. The procedure involves making a transverse cut in the proximal tibial metaphysis and removing a wedge of bone or opening the cut in a wedge-shaped fashion and packing it with bone graft to change the geometry of the lower limb to unload the affected condyle. Rehabilitation is comparatively long with HTO, with bracing locked in full extension and ambulation with crutches for the first 6 weeks after surgery while the osteotomy site heals. Rehabilitation to regain functional flexion and good quadriceps tone should be continued while the osteotomy site is healing and may take 6 months to 1 year after surgery. The indications for tibial osteotomy are similar to those for osteoarthritis, including early degenerative changes isolated to a single compartment without the presence of late-stage degenerative disease.

Koshino[18] described the results of HTO on 37 knees with spontaneous ON (35 cases in the medial compartment, 2 cases in the lateral compartment) at 62 months of mean follow-up (range: 24–102 months). He reported better postoperative clinical outcomes, measured using the Knee Society Scoring System, in patients with earlier stage disease (scores of 95 ± 2, 90 ± 7, and 81 ± 11 points in patients with stage II, stage III, and stage IV disease, respectively).

Unicompartmental knee arthroplasty

Patients with single compartment degenerative changes who do not qualify for osteochondral transfer or HTO can be treated with unicompartmental knee arthroplasty. This procedure involves replacement of only the diseased femoral condyle and the associated tibial articular surface, as shown in **Fig. 9**. In contrast to a complete bicondylar TKA, this procedure provides the benefit of minimizing the incision size and the loss of native bone stock. Some researchers report a shorter rehabilitation period and less postoperative pain than after TKA, allowing for future revision as necessary.[36–39] Because SPONK is typically a unicondylar disease that does not progress to the second condyle, unicompartmental arthroplasty is an appropriate choice for treatment in most patients whose degenerative changes are limited to a single condyle.

A recent meta-analysis of results from five reports for unicompartmental arthroplasty for SPONK reported 90% good outcomes, 16% poor outcomes, and 13% revisions in 64 knees over a mean follow-up of 5 years.[40] When only knees

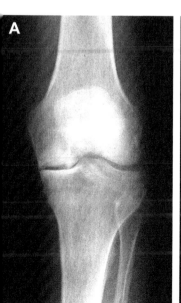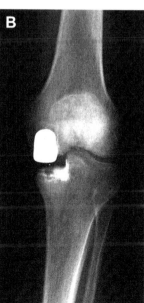

Fig. 9. Stage 4 SPONK (A) treated with unicompartmental knee arthroplasty (B).

operated on after 1985 were considered, the rate of good outcomes was 100%, although the cohort size was only 10 patients. Myers and colleagues[40] attribute this improvement in outcomes to the widespread adoption of modern cementing techniques in all knees with ON after 1985.

Total knee arthroplasty

In some patients, TKA may be an appropriate choice of treatment. Because TKA replaces the patient's femoral and tibial articular surfaces, and optionally the patellar surface, patients who have late-stage arthritis that has progressed to involvement of all compartments are appropriate candidates.

Outcomes for TKA are similar to those found for osteoarthritis. In the previously mentioned meta-analysis, 148 patients who underwent TKA for SPONK had a good outcome rate of 92%, with a poor outcome rate of 6% and a revision rate of 3% at a mean follow-up of 4 years (range not reported).[40] When only the 23 TKAs performed after 1985 were considered, all had good clinical outcomes.

SECONDARY OSTEONECROSIS

Secondary ON of the knee is a debilitating condition that often presents with mild or nonspecific symptoms in the early stages. However, in the later stages, the joint collapses, leading to the need for joint replacement for disabling pain. ON can affect any of the large joints, although the knee is the second most commonly affected site, with an incidence of approximately 10% of that for the hip.[41]

Secondary ON differs from SPONK, as can be compared in **Table 1**. The usual presentation is of bilateral knee disease in younger patients (<55 years of age) affecting both condyles with multiple lesions, as illustrated in **Fig. 10**. Patients typically have involvement of other large joints, especially the hip. With the incidence of secondary ON of the hip representing 90% of all large joints combined, much of what is understood about the pathology, pathophysiology, and risk factors for disease of the knee has been extrapolated from hip reports.

Etiology, Pathology, and Pathogenesis

The pathology of ON is similar in all cases irrespective of the cause. The size and location of the lesion typically influence the rate of disease progression. In some cases, small lesions may stabilize spontaneously,[42] but in more than 90% of cases, the lesions progress. Ischemia and necrosis prevent repair in a wedge- or cone-shaped region and limit repair at its periphery, causing bone resorption and replacement with fibrous

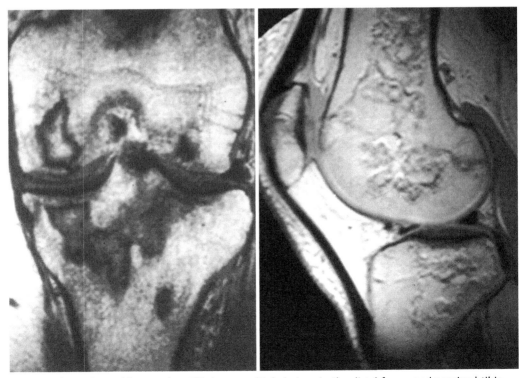

Fig. 10. MRI of a patient with secondary ON shows multiple lesions in the distal femur and proximal tibia.

and granulation tissue. This acellular region weakens the mechanical stability of the surrounding bone, leading to subchondral fracture, cartilage degeneration, and eventual collapse of the affected condyle or condyles. The degenerated or collapsed regions place additional stress on their adjacent articular surfaces, inducing further degenerative changes.

ON seems to have multiple etiologies that, in some cases, are additive to create bone conditions marked by elevated intraosseous pressure or circulatory disruption, eventually leading to focal ischemia and necrosis.

It is postulated that corticosteroid use and alcohol consumption increase intraosseous adipocyte size and proliferation, displacing the bone marrow.[43–45] With bone being a nonexpansile compartment, this causes increased intraosseous pressure and eventual vascular collapse and ischemia. Several other factors associated with ON are believed to increase intraosseous pressure. Gaucher's disease, leukemia, and other myeloproliferative disorders are all similarly associated with bone marrow displacement and increased compartment pressure.

Other associated factors are believed to lead to ON through direct restriction or occlusion of blood vessels. Emboli composed of fat sickled red blood cells, or nitrogen bubbles (as in caisson decompression sickness, or caisson disease), may directly mechanically occlude vessels, producing ischemia. Smoking is known to cause vasoconstriction, further promoting ischemia. Thrombophilia and hypofibrinolysis have also been associated with development of ON.

Indirect factors, with poorly understood mechanisms of action, have also been associated with ON. Systemic lupus erythematosus has a well-reported association with ON,[46,47] and several genetic risk factors have been reported.[48] For example, a mutation of type II collagen has been identified in three families with autosomal dominant inheritance of ON.[49]

Diagnostic Methods

Patients who have ON usually present with knee pain of gradual onset located over the medial or lateral condyle, or both, depending on the distribution of the necrotic foci. Most patients have a history of one or more associated risk factors, with corticosteroid use and systemic lupus erythematosus being the most common.[25] Secondary ON of the knee can be difficult to diagnose because the pain can be mistaken for a meniscal or ligamentous injury in the knee. The pain can also be misinterpreted as referred from the hips because

many patients with secondary ON of the knee also have disease in those joints. Because of these diagnostic difficulties, obtaining bilateral AP and lateral radiographs, in addition to MRI, of all symptomatic joints in patients with risk factors for secondary ON is important to make the earliest diagnosis. Radionucleotide bone scanning has traditionally been recommended as a diagnostic tool for secondary ON, especially in early stages of the disease. However, in a recent report by Mont and colleagues,[17] bone scanning detected only 37 (64%) of 53 lesions in patients with symptomatic ON of the knee, whereas MRI detected all 53 lesions (100%). Based on the low sensitivity reported in that study, and on the possibility of normal scans during the ischemic phase of the disease, the authors do not recommend bone scanning as a diagnostic tool for ON of the knee or other joints.

Secondary ON lesions progress to collapse in a similar manner to those of SPONK and are staged using the same modified Ficat and Arlet system previously described and shown in **Table 2**. Sizing is performed using the systems developed by Aglietti and colleagues[23] and Mont and colleagues,[25] as shown in **Figs. 5** and **6**. Unlike SPONK, multiple lesions can occur in secondary ON and can be found in the epiphysis, diaphysis, or metaphysis of the femur or tibia, or both. To assist in the description of the extent of disease, lesions can be localized using the system described by Mont and colleagues,[25] as shown in **Fig. 11**.

Treatment for Secondary Osteonecrosis

There are multiple treatment options available for secondary ON, ranging from joint-preserving techniques to total joint arthroplasties, with their use based on the different stages and sizes of the lesions. Although some of the treatments overlap with those described for SPONK, the indications, effectiveness, and potential pitfalls often differ. **Fig. 12** illustrates the treatment protocol used by the authors for secondary ON, which includes the methods of treatment described in this section.

Nonoperative treatment

Historically, nonoperative options for the treatment of ON consist of protected weight bearing, with analgesics as required for pain. The rationale was to limit stress on the affected joint long enough for physiologic healing of the lesion to take place. This approach may be indicated for asymptomatic patients and as an initial treatment for patients who present with stage I to III lesions without severe symptoms. Unfortunately, the effectiveness of this treatment method is limited,

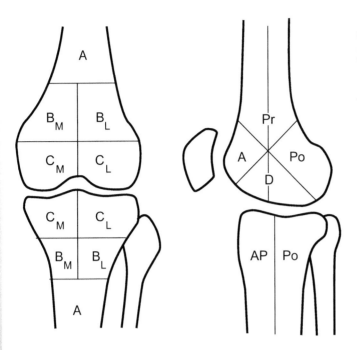

Fig. 11. To assist in localization of the lesion, the distal femur and proximal tibia are divided into four quadrants each on the AP radiograph. On the lateral radiograph, the femur is divided into anterior (A), posterior (Po), proximal (Pr), and distal (D) quadrants and the tibia is divided into anterior and posterior columns. (*Adapted from* Mont MA, Baumgarten KM, Rifai A, et al. Atraumatic osteonecrosis of the knee. J Bone Joint Surg Am 2000;82:1281; with permission.)

with only 20% of patients in one study having a good clinical outcome without requiring surgery after minimum 2-year follow-up.[25] The authors do not advocate this method.

More recently, various pharmacologic agents have been proposed or tried for the treatment of ON of the femoral head. These have included the use of bisphosphonates, lipid-lowering agents, and anticoagulants.[50–53] Although used to attempt to treat hip disease, they have not specifically been used for knee ON but might be applied for treatment in the future.

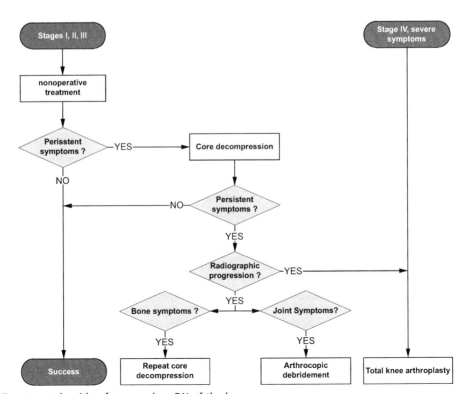

Fig. 12. Treatment algorithm for secondary ON of the knee.

Core decompression

Core decompression is a minimally traumatic procedure that can be performed on an outpatient basis. Traditional core decompression techniques involved the drilling of a single track to the affected subchondral region using a trephine 6 to 10 mm in diameter through an extra-articular approach, with optional filling of the defect with bone graft. This procedure relieves the regionally elevated intra-osseous pressure in the bone compartment. Some investigators believe that this may improve circulation and facilitate the physiologic healing process. Core decompression could be effective in preventing disease progression if performed before condylar collapse. In one study, 73% of patients treated with traditional core decompression for Ficat and Arlet stage I to III disease had good to excellent results at a mean follow-up of 11 years (range: 4–16 years), as defined by a Knee Society Score of 80 points or higher.[21]

Since 2000, the senior author (MAM) has been utilizing a percutaneous drilling technique using multiple passes with a small-diameter (3.2 mm) drill bit under fluoroscopic guidance, as shown in **Fig. 13**, performed on an outpatient basis. This technique reduces morbidity and improves outcomes by reducing structural compromise of the bone and permitting immediate mobilization after surgery. Marulanda and colleagues[54] reported on a series of 61 knees with Ficat and Arlet stage I and II secondary ON of the knee treated with percutaneous core decompression. Fifty-six knees (92%) had good to excellent outcomes, defined as a Knee Society Score of 80 points or greater and no progression to TKA at a mean follow-up of 37 months (range: 24–50 months).

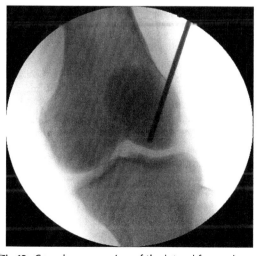

Fig. 13. Core decompression of the lateral femoral condyle using an extra-articular approach with a small-diameter drill bit.

Core decompression with arthroscopic assistance

Core decompression with arthroscopic assistance may be an appropriate treatment in patients who have persistent symptoms after initial core decompression. Diagnostic arthroscopy is performed as part of the procedure to visualize any chondral lesions or defects directly and to identify any other intra-articular pathologic conditions that could be responsible for the patient's symptoms (ie, torn meniscus). Therapeutic arthroscopic procedures, such as débridement or meniscectomy, can be performed on any identified intra-articular pathologic finding, or the procedure can be converted to open treatment, such as an OATS procedure, if appropriate based on the results of the arthroscopic exploration (focal cartilage defect found). Core decompression can then be performed as part of the same procedure.

Miller and colleagues[55] reported a case series detailing symptomatic improvement in patients treated with arthroscopic débridement of necrotic lesions but also concluded that this treatment does not alter the course of the disease. Ruch and Satterfield[56] reported that in a series of 95 arthroscopically assisted core decompressions of the hip, 10% of patients with collapsed femoral heads also had an associated labral tear that could be responsible for their symptoms. The authors are not aware of similar reports for the knee but have discovered and treated several meniscal tears in their own patient group, with symptomatic improvement.

Bone grafting

Various bone grafting techniques have been reported for the treatment of osteochondral defects and collapsed lesions of the femoral condyles in secondary ON. These procedures are performed to restore the structural integrity of condylar bone and restore chondral continuity of the articular surface, with the goal of preventing or delaying condylar degeneration to the stage at which knee arthroplasty becomes the only viable treatment.

Fukui and colleagues[57] treated 10 knees with autogenous osteoperiosteal grafts harvested from the iliac crest, with the curvature of the harvested segment matched to approximate the contour of the defect. Nine of the 10 knees had significant clinical improvement at a mean follow-up of 79 months (range: 31–158 months), with no salvage procedures necessary. Rijnen and colleagues[58] treated 8 knees with bone impaction grafting, débriding the necrotic tissue through an extra-articular bone window and filling the defect with impacted autogenous trabecular bone chips. Six of 8 knees achieved a minimum Knee Society Score of

80 points with no revisions at a mean follow-up of 51 months (range: 29–93 months). Flynn and colleagues[59] treated eight patients with secondary ON of the knee with autologous osteochondral grafting, with six having good or excellent clinical results (rated on a custom scale reported by these researchers), at a mean follow-up of 55 months (range: 24–109 months). Meyers and colleagues[60] treated 3 knees with osteochondral grafts, with excellent clinical results (18 points on the Merle d'Aubigné and Postel scale as modified by these investigators) in all knees (2 knees at 3 years of follow-up and 1 knee at 4 years of follow-up).

Unfortunately, studies of bone grafting for secondary ON of the knee are limited to a few retrospective reports, with small patient groups in all cases. However, given the limited alternative joint-preserving treatments available and the relatively young age of many patients, bone grafting may be a useful treatment method in carefully selected patients with intact articular cartilage.

Total knee arthroplasty

Unicondylar prostheses are contraindicated in patients with secondary ON of the knee because of frequent multicondylar involvement. TKA is indicated in patients who have stage IV disease, with lesions on both sides of the joint and collapsed articular cartilage. At this stage of disease progression, prosthetic implantation is currently the only viable means of restoring joint anatomy and providing symptomatic and functional improvement.

A meta-analysis of published results for TKA for secondary ON revealed only 74% good outcomes, with a 20% revision rate in 150 patients at a mean follow-up of 8 years (range: 4.2–10 years).[40] When only arthroplasties performed after 1985 were considered, good outcomes occurred in 97% of cases. The significant improvement in results in later-performed arthroplasties is believed to be a consequence of the use of cemented components for all patients who had ON and the use of ancillary stems in patients with severe metaphyseal or diaphyseal lesions, or otherwise compromised bone strength, to ensure optimal fixation and stability of the prostheses.[61]

POSTARTHROSCOPIC OSTEONECROSIS

Arthroscopy has evolved to become one of the most commonly performed orthopedic procedures today. ON of the knee has been described as an infrequent but often destructive complication of arthroscopic surgery, with approximately 70 cases reported to date.[62,63]

Etiology, Pathology, and Pathogenesis

Postarthroscopic ON of the knee has been described in several reports, developing after arthroscopic meniscectomy, shaver-assisted chondroplasty, anterior cruciate ligament reconstruction, and laser- or radiofrequency-assisted débridement. It usually affects the epiphyseal region of a single condyle in the operated knee and has been reported to develop at a mean time of approximately 24 weeks after surgery (range: 4–92 weeks).[62] On rare occasions, concurrent lesions have been reported in a femoral condyle and an adjacent tibial plateau, in addition to in the patella.[64] Further characteristics of this condition can be reviewed in **Table 1**.

The pathophysiology of osteonecrosis following these procedures is not completely understood. However, a recent study of histopathological samples from eight patients who developed osteonecrosis after arthroscopic meniscectomy without laser or radiofrequency assistance provided evidence that subchondral fracture is the primary event confirming similar findings from an earlier case report.[63,65] Some researchers have suggested that postarthroscopic ON may be the result of insufficiency fractures or microfractures, noting changes in weight distribution and an increase in tibiofemoral contact pressure after meniscal tear or meniscectomy.[66–68] Some lesions in ON after meniscectomy have been noted to bear a strong similarity to SPONK lesions in histologic and radiographic appearance, with dead bone found only distally to a subchondral fracture, and in clinical presentation and course, suggesting that this condition may not be true ON in some cases.[63,69]

It has been proposed that laser- or radiofrequency-assisted arthroscopic surgery may produce ON through direct thermal injury or through photoacoustic shock.[64,70,71] Thermal damage to subchondral bone may lead to an inflammatory response causing bone edema, ischemia, and eventual necrosis. Photoacoustic shock is caused by the rapid vaporization of cellular contents and intracellular water, with the expanding gases producing a shock wave that penetrates and damages subchondral bone, leading to an inflammatory response with eventual edema and necrosis. The appearance of these lesions on MRI has been reported to be consistent with ON, and histologic samples taken from two patients in one published case report revealed large areas of ON, suggesting that the condition in these cases was true secondary ON from the thermal injury or photoacoustic shock.[64,72]

Considering the current knowledge regarding postarthroscopic ON, it seems that this diagnosis may, in fact, represent two distinct conditions with different etiologies and pathophysiologic findings. In some cases, the condition may not be true ON but rather a postarthroscopic form of SPONK, with subchondral fracture secondary to altered bone loading, resulting in ischemia of the distal fracture fragment. In other cases, the condition may be the direct result of a thermal or photoacoustic shock injury caused by laser or radiofrequency surgical tools, resulting in subchondral bone marrow edema, with resulting ischemia and necrosis. Further investigations are required to clarify the precise pathophysiology of these injuries.

Diagnostic Methods

Patients with postarthroscopic ON usually present with acute-onset or worsening of knee pain and a recent history of therapeutic arthroscopic surgery. Because most of these patients have undergone arthroscopic surgery for knee pain, the pain associated with this ON may be mistaken for failed treatment or a return of the original injury. AP and lateral radiographs, in addition to MRI scans, should be obtained for the symptomatic joint. Staging and sizing can be performed using the modified Ficat and Arlet system,[19–21] or the system of Motohashi and colleagues,[22] Aglietti and colleagues,[23] or Mont and colleagues,[25] as previously described and illustrated in **Figs. 5, 6,** and **11**.

Treatment of Postarthroscopic Osteonecrosis of the Knee

Because of the relatively recent characterization of this condition and the low incidence, there is little published information about its treatment. As a result, treatment results for SPONK and secondary ON, in addition to individual case reports, have been used to guide decision making.

Nonoperative treatment

Initial treatment for postarthroscopic ON is nonsurgical, with protected weight bearing and analgesics as required. The rationale for this approach is similar to that in the treatment of SPONK and secondary ON. Restricted loading and stress on the affected condyle may improve physiologic healing by minimizing additional or ongoing stress and trauma. Individual cases of resolution of symptoms and return to predisease function have been reported with nonoperative treatment, but the authors are not aware of any published results assessing the effectiveness of this treatment for postarthroscopic ON.[64,73] Extrapolating from results and experience with SPONK and secondary ON, it is expected that nonoperative treatment has the best chance for success in patients

presenting with small, early-stage, precollapse lesions without degenerative articular surface changes.

Joint-preserving surgical treatment

Patients who fail nonoperative treatment may benefit from core decompression or HTO, two joint-preserving treatments shown to be effective in some patients with SPONK or secondary ON. Garino and colleagues[64] reported two cases of postarthroscopic ON treated with core decompression, although both patients ultimately went on to further surgical treatment. One patient was treated with core decompression of the medial femoral condyle and percutaneous drilling of the medial femoral condyle and medial tibial plateau for late-stage SPONK with a grade IV lesion of the articular cartilage (grading system not specified but presumed to be the International Cartilage Repair Society system). This patient was then treated with unicompartmental knee arthroplasty 1 year after decompression and drilling, with a reported good early result (no evaluation system or follow-up time specified). The second patient was treated with drilling of the patella using an anterior approach for suspected ON after laser-assisted chondroplasty of the patella and medial femoral condyle. One year after this procedure, the patient was treated with a patellectomy, with reported resolution of the pain (no pain level evaluation system or follow-up time reported). Nevertheless, because patients being considered for core decompression have already failed nonoperative treatment, the authors believe that core decompression may be indicated before considering more invasive surgical treatments.

Carefully selected patients who fail nonoperative treatment and core decompression may be candidates for treatment with HTO. Indications are similar as for patients with osteoarthritis, including younger patients with unicondylar disease and early degenerative changes without late-stage disease. Johnson and colleagues[73] have reported two cases of HTO used to treat ON after arthroscopic partial medial meniscectomy, with one performed at 8 months after arthroscopic surgery and the other at 10 months after arthroscopic surgery. However, these investigators did not report any clinical results or follow-up time for these patients.

Knee arthroplasty

Patients who fail joint-preserving treatments or are not candidates for these procedures because of advanced disease with collapsed articular cartilage should be treated with unicompartmental or TKA. Unicompartmental knee arthroplasty is an appropriate choice of treatment in patients with disease limited to a single compartment, preserving as much of the patient's native bone as possible. Patients with involvement of multiple compartments should be treated with a TKA, as shown in **Fig. 14**.

Bonutti and colleagues[62] treated 19 patients diagnosed with postarthroscopic ON with minimally invasive knee arthroplasty, performing 4 unicompartmental arthroplasties and 15 tricompartmental arthroplasties. Clinical outcomes were determined using the Knee Society rating system. Eighteen patients had good or excellent clinical outcomes (defined as a Knee Society score of 80 points or greater), with a mean score of 92 points (range: 60–100 points) at a mean follow-up of 62 months

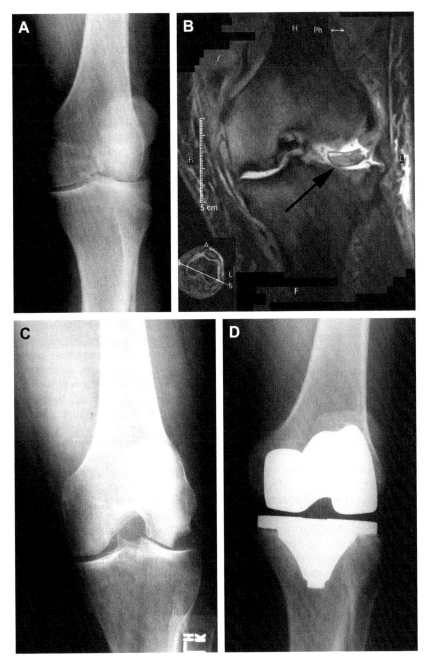

Fig. 14. A patient complaining of a locking knee (*A*) underwent arthroscopic radiofrequency-assisted chondroplasty and partial meniscectomy. Subsequently, he developed postarthroscopic ON of the lateral femoral condyle, visible on MRI (*B, arrow*) 2 months after surgery (note detached condylar fragment). (*C*) Marked degeneration of the lateral condyle was visible on a radiograph 4 months after surgery. (*D*) This patient later underwent TKA.

(range: 24–133 months). The one patient with a poor outcome received a tricompartmental prosthesis and had her walking ability limited by unexplained moderate pain despite good radiographic alignment. Postoperative standing radiographs showed a mean alignment of 5° of valgus (range: 3°–8°), with no change in alignment and no impending radiographic failures or progressive radiolucencies at the time of final follow-up. There have been several other case reports and case series of unicompartmental arthroplasty or TKA used as a definitive treatment in patients with postarthroscopic ON of the knee refractory to joint-preserving treatment.[63,64,72,73,74] None of the researchers reported unsuccessful outcomes with knee arthroplasty, but in all cases, little or no data were provided about the patients' clinical outcomes. Nevertheless, based on all the available results, minimally invasive knee arthroplasty is believed to be an excellent treatment option for postarthroscopic ON.

SUMMARY

ON of the knee refers to three distinct disorders: SPONK, secondary ON of the knee, and postarthroscopic ON of the knee. These conditions can be clearly distinguished from each other based on patient demographics, condylar involvement, number and distribution of lesions, and the presence or absence of several associated risk factors. Plain radiographs and MRI can assist in distinguishing these disorders and aid in planning treatment. Several joint-preserving surgical treatments (including arthroscopy, osteochondral defect repair, core decompression, nonvascular bone grafting, and HTO) have been used in selected patients. When an appropriate implant is selected, unicompartmental (for SPONK only) and total knee (for secondary ON) arthroplasty has shown excellent results in patients with late degenerative changes.

REFERENCES

1. Ahlbäck S, Bauer GC, Bohne WH. Spontaneous osteonecrosis of the knee. Arthritis Rheum 1968; 11:705–33.
2. Yamamoto T, Bullough PG. Spontaneous osteonecrosis of the knee: the result of subchondral insufficiency fracture. J Bone Joint Surg Am 2000;82: 858–66.
3. Narvaez JA, Narvaez J, De Lama E, et al. Spontaneous osteonecrosis of the knee associated with tibial plateau and femoral condyle insufficiency stress fracture. Eur Radiol 2003;13:1843–8.
4. Kattapuram TM, Kattapuram SV. Spontaneous osteonecrosis of the knee. Eur J Radiol 2008;67:42–8.
5. Takeda M, Higuchi H, Kimura M, et al. Spontaneous osteonecrosis of the knee: histopathological differences between early and progressive cases. J Bone Joint Surg Br 2008;90:324–9.
6. Kantor H. Bone marrow pressure in osteonecrosis of the femoral condyle (Ahlbäck's disease). Arch Orthop Trauma Surg 1987;106:349–52.
7. Arnoldi CC, Lemperg K, Linderholm H. Intraosseous hypertension and pain in the knee. J Bone Joint Surg Br 1975;57:360–3.
8. Mears SC, Mont MA, Jones LC, et al. Osteonecrosis of the knee. Washington, DC: AAOS; 2005.
9. Geusens P, Dinant G. Integrating a gender dimension into osteoporosis and fracture risk research. Gend Med 2007;4(Suppl B):S147–61.
10. Ohdera T, Miyagi S, Tokunaga M, et al. Spontaneous osteonecrosis of the lateral femoral condyle of the knee: a report of 11 cases. Arch Orthop Trauma Surg 2008; 128(8):825–31.
11. Schindler OS, Misra R, Spalding TJ. Osteonecrosis of the medial tibial plateau: a case report. J Orthop Surg (Hong Kong) 2006;14:325–9.
12. Soucacos PN, Johnson EO, Soultanis K, et al. Diagnosis and management of the osteonecrotic triad of the knee. Orthop Clin North Am 2004;35:371–81, x.
13. Pollack MS, Dalinka MK, Kressel HY, et al. Magnetic resonance imaging in the evaluation of suspected osteonecrosis of the knee. Skeletal Radiol 1987;16: 121–7.
14. Greyson ND, Lotem MM, Gross AE, et al. Radionuclide evaluation of spontaneous femoral osteonecrosis. Radiology 1982;142:729–35.
15. al-Rowaih A, Wingstrand H, Lindstrand A, et al. Three-phase scintimetry in osteonecrosis of the knee. Acta Orthop Scand 1990;61:120–7.
16. Rozing PM, Insall J, Bohne WH. Spontaneous osteonecrosis of the knee. J Bone Joint Surg Am 1980;62:2–7.
17. Mont MA, Ulrich SD, Seyler TM, et al. Bone scanning of limited value for diagnosis of symptomatic oligofocal and multifocal osteonecrosis. J Rheumatol 2008; 35(8):1629–34.
18. Koshino T. The treatment of spontaneous osteonecrosis of the knee by high tibial osteotomy with and without bone-grafting or drilling of the lesion. J Bone Joint Surg Am 1982;64:47–58.
19. Ficat RP, Arlet J. Functional investigation of bone under normal conditions. In: Hungerford D, editor. Ischemia and necrosis of bone. Baltimore (MD): Williams and Wilkins; 1980. p. 29–52.
20. Ficat RP. Idiopathic bone necrosis of the femoral head. Early diagnosis and treatment. J Bone Joint Surg Br 1985;67:3–9.
21. Mont MA, Tomek IM, Hungerford DS. Core decompression for avascular necrosis of the distal femur: long term followup. Clin Orthop Relat Res 1997;334:124–30.
22. Motohashi M, Morii T, Koshino T. Clinical course and roentgenographic changes of osteonecrosis in the

femoral condyle under conservative treatment. Clin Orthop Relat Res 1991;266:156–61.

23. Aglietti P, Insall JN, Buzzi R, et al. Idiopathic osteonecrosis of the knee. Aetiology, prognosis and treatment. J Bone Joint Surg Br 1983;65:588–97.

24. Kerboul M, Thomine J, Postel M, et al. The conservative surgical treatment of idiopathic aseptic necrosis of the femoral head. J Bone Joint Surg Br 1974;56:291–6.

25. Mont MA, Baumgarten KM, Rifai A, et al. Atraumatic osteonecrosis of the knee. J Bone Joint Surg Am 2000;82:1279–90.

26. Uchio Y, Ochi M, Adachi N, et al. Effectiveness of an insole with a lateral wedge for idiopathic osteonecrosis of the knee. J Bone Joint Surg Br 2000;82:724–7.

27. Lotke PA, Abend JA, Ecker ML. The treatment of osteonecrosis of the medial femoral condyle. Clin Orthop Relat Res 1982;171:109–16.

28. Yates PJ, Calder JD, Stranks GJ, et al. Early MRI diagnosis and non-surgical management of spontaneous osteonecrosis of the knee. Knee 2007;14:112–6.

29. Steadman JR, Rodkey WG, Briggs KK. Microfracture to treat full-thickness chondral defects: surgical technique, rehabilitation, and outcomes. J Knee Surg 2002;15:170–6.

30. Akgun I, Kesmezacar H, Ogut T, et al. Arthroscopic microfracture treatment for osteonecrosis of the knee. Arthroscopy 2005;21:834–43.

31. Gudas R, Kalesinskas RJ, Kimtys V, et al. A prospective randomized clinical study of mosaic osteochondral autologous transplantation versus microfracture for the treatment of osteochondral defects in the knee joint in young athletes. Arthroscopy 2005;21:1066–75.

32. Gudas R, Stankevicius E, Monastyreckiene E, et al. Osteochondral autologous transplantation versus microfracture for the treatment of articular cartilage defects in the knee joint in athletes. Knee Surg Sports Traumatol Arthrosc 2006;14:834–42.

33. Hangody L, Kish G, Karpati Z, et al. Arthroscopic autogenous osteochondral mosaicplasty for the treatment of femoral condylar articular defects. A preliminary report. Knee Surg Sports Traumatol Arthrosc 1997;5:262–7.

34. Hangody L, Vasarhelyi G, Hangody LR, et al. Autologous osteochondral grafting—technique and long-term results. Injury 2008;39(Suppl 1):S32–9.

35. Forst J, Forst R, Heller KD, et al. Spontaneous osteonecrosis of the femoral condyle: causal treatment by early core decompression. Arch Orthop Trauma Surg 1998;117:18–22.

36. Springer BD, Scott RD, Thornhill TS. Conversion of failed unicompartmental knee arthroplasty to TKA. Clin Orthop Relat Res 2006;446:214–20.

37. Newman JH, Ackroyd CE, Shah NA. Unicompartmental or total knee replacement? Five-year results of a prospective, randomised trial of 102 osteoarthritic knees with unicompartmental arthritis. J Bone Joint Surg Br 1998;80:862–5.

38. Levine WN, Ozuna RM, Scott RD, et al. Conversion of failed modern unicompartmental arthroplasty to total knee arthroplasty. J Arthroplasty 1996;11: 797–801.

39. Barrett WP, Scott RD. Revision of failed unicondylar unicompartmental knee arthroplasty. J Bone Joint Surg Am 1987;69:1328–35.

40. Myers TG, Cui Q, Kuskowski M, et al. Outcomes of total and unicompartmental knee arthroplasty for secondary and spontaneous osteonecrosis of the knee. J Bone Joint Surg Am 2006;88(Suppl 3): 76–82.

41. Mankin HJ. Nontraumatic necrosis of bone (osteonecrosis). N Engl J Med 1992;326:1473–9.

42. Cheng EY, Thongtrangan I, Laorr A, et al. Spontaneous resolution of osteonecrosis of the femoral head. J Bone Joint Surg Am 2004;86:2594–9.

43. Lee MS, Hsieh PH, Chang YH, et al. Elevated intraosseous pressure in the intertrochanteric region is associated with poorer results in osteonecrosis of the femoral head treated by multiple drilling. J Bone Joint Surg Br 2008;90:852–7.

44. Mont MA, Carbone JJ, Fairbank AC. Core decompression versus nonoperative management for osteonecrosis of the hip. Clin Orthop Relat Res 1996;324:169–78.

45. Miyanishi K, Yamamoto T, Irisa T, et al. Bone marrow fat cell enlargement and a rise in intraosseous pressure in steroid-treated rabbits with osteonecrosis. Bone 2002;30:185–90.

46. Abeles M, Urman JD, Rothfield NF. Aseptic necrosis of bone in systemic lupus erythematosus. Relationship to corticosteroid therapy. Arch Intern Med 1978;138:750–4.

47. Zizic TM, Marcoux C, Hungerford DS, et al. Corticosteroid therapy associated with ischemic necrosis of bone in systemic lupus erythematosus. Am J Med 1985;79:596–604.

48. Mont MA, Hungerford DS. Osteonecrosis of the shoulder, knee, and ankle. In: Urbaniak JR, Jones JP, editors. Osteonecrosis: etiology, diagnosis, and treatment. Rosemont (IL): American Academy of Orothopaedic Surgeons; 1997. p. 429–36.

49. Liu YF, Chen WM, Lin YF, et al. Type II collagen gene variants and inherited osteonecrosis of the femoral head. N Engl J Med 2005;352(22):2294–301.

50. Agarwala S, Jain D, Joshi VR, et al. Efficacy of alendronate, a bisphosphonate, in the treatment of AVN of the hip. A prospective open-label study. Rheumatology (Oxford) 2005;44:352–9.

51. Lai KA, Shen WJ, Yang CY, et al. The use of alendronate to prevent early collapse of the femoral head in patients with nontraumatic osteonecrosis. A randomized clinical study. J Bone Joint Surg Am 2005;87:2155–9.

52. Ramachandran M, Ward K, Brown RR, et al. Intravenous bisphosphonate therapy for traumatic

osteonecrosis of the femoral head in adolescents. J Bone Joint Surg Am 2007;89:1727–34.

53. Pritchett JW. Statin therapy decreases the risk of osteonecrosis in patients receiving steroids. Clin Orthop Relat Res 2001;386:173–8.

54. Marulanda G, Seyler TM, Sheikh NH, et al. Percutaneous drilling for the treatment of secondary osteonecrosis of the knee. J Bone Joint Surg Br 2006;88:740–6.

55. Miller GK, Maylahn DJ, Drennan DB. The treatment of idiopathic osteonecrosis of the medial femoral condyle with arthroscopic debridement. Arthroscopy 1986;2:21–9.

56. Ruch DS, Satterfield W. The use of arthroscopy to document accurate position of core decompression of the hip. Arthroscopy 1998;14:617–9.

57. Fukui N, Kurosawa H, Kawakami A, et al. Iliac bone graft for steroid-associated osteonecrosis of the femoral condyle. Clin Orthop Relat Res 2002;401:185–93.

58. Rijnen WH, Luttjeboer JS, Schreurs BW, et al. Bone impaction grafting for corticosteroid-associated osteonecrosis of the knee. J Bone Joint Surg Am 2006;88(Suppl 3):62–8.

59. Flynn JM, Springfield DS, Mankin HJ. Osteoarticular allografts to treat distal femoral osteonecrosis. Clin Orthop Relat Res 1994;303:38–43.

60. Meyers MH, Akeson W, Convery FR. Resurfacing of the knee with fresh osteochondral allograft. J Bone Joint Surg Am 1989;71:704–13.

61. Mont MA, Rifai A, Baumgarten KM, et al. Total knee arthroplasty for osteonecrosis. J Bone Joint Surg Am 2002;84:599–603.

62. Bonutti PM, Seyler TM, Delanois RE, et al. Osteonecrosis of the knee after laser or radiofrequency-assisted arthroscopy: treatment with minimally invasive knee arthroplasty. J Bone Joint Surg Am 2006;88(Suppl 3):69–75.

63. MacDessi SJ, Brophy RH, Bullough PG, et al. Subchondral fracture following arthroscopic knee surgery. A series of eight cases. J Bone Joint Surg Am 2008;90:1007–12.

64. Garino JP, Lotke PA, Sapega AA, et al. Osteonecrosis of the knee following laser-assisted arthroscopic surgery: a report of six cases. Arthroscopy 1995;11:467–74.

65. Nakamura N, Horibe S, Nakamura S, et al. Subchondral microfracture of the knee without osteonecrosis after arthroscopic medial meniscectomy. Arthroscopy 2002;18:538–41.

66. Brahme SK, Fox JM, Ferkel RD, et al. Osteonecrosis of the knee after arthroscopic surgery: diagnosis with MR imaging. Radiology 1991;178:851–3.

67. Norman A, Baker ND. Spontaneous osteonecrosis of the knee and medial meniscal tears. Radiology 1978;129:653–6.

68. Krause WR, Pope MH, Johnson RJ, et al. Mechanical changes in the knee after meniscectomy. J Bone Joint Surg Am 1976;58:599–604.

69. Pape D, Seil R, Anagnostakos K, et al. Postarthroscopic osteonecrosis of the knee. Arthroscopy 2007;23:428–38.

70. Lee EW, Paulos LE, Warren RF. Complications of thermal energy in knee surgery—part II. Clin Sports Med 2002;21:753–63.

71. Dew DK. Laser biophysics for the orthopaedic surgeon. Clin Orthop Relat Res 1995;310:6–13.

72. Janzen DL, Kosarek FJ, Helms CA, et al. Osteonecrosis after contact neodymium:yttrium aluminum garnet arthroscopic laser meniscectomy. AJR Am J Roentgenol 1997;169:855–8.

73. Johnson TC, Evans JA, Gilley JA, et al. Osteonecrosis of the knee after arthroscopic surgery for meniscal tears and chondral lesions. Arthroscopy 2000;16:254–61.

74. Prues-Latour V, Bonvin JC, Fritschy D. Nine cases of osteonecrosis in elderly patients following arthroscopic meniscectomy. Knee Surg Sports Traumatol Arthrosc 1998;6:142–7.

Cellular-Based Therapy for Osteonecrosis

Valérie Gangji, MD, PhD[a],*, Jean-Philippe Hauzeur, MD, PhD[b]

KEYWORDS

- Osteonecrosis • Bone marrow • Stem cell
- Cellular therapy

Nontraumatic osteonecrosis (ON) of the femoral head is a painful disorder of the hip most commonly associated with corticosteroid therapy and alcohol abuse, which often leads in its final stage to femoral head collapse and subsequent total hip arthroplasty.[1] Various efforts have been made to enhance the healing of osteonecrotic sequestrum before collapse occurs because total hip arthroplasty is a less than optimal option in young patients. Although different pathophysiologic mechanisms leading to ischemia have been postulated for this disease, none can explain the insufficient bone repair following the occurrence of the lesion and its evolution to bone collapse. Hernigou colleagues[2] were among the first to suggest that ON might also be a disease of bone cells or mesenchymal stem cells. The levels of activity and the number of mesenchymal stem cells in the hematopoietic and the stromal compartments of the bone marrow have been shown to be depressed in patients with ON of the femoral head,[3] as well as the capacity of proliferation of osteoblastic cells.[4] These findings raise the possibility of a pathophysiologic approach to ON treatment by implantation into the necrotic lesion of stem cells from mesenchymal tissues including bone obtained after autologous bone marrow concentration.[5,6]

This review article describes bone remodeling in the context of ON as a bone disease, the use of stem cells in bone and vascular diseases, and cellular therapy in ON.

BONE REMODELING

The skeleton is an extremely dynamic tissue at the microscopic level in being able to sustain the tremendous loads placed on it in everyday life which depends on, among other factors, being able to remodel and repair the constant microcracks or lesions that develop within the bone. The fundamental mechanisms of bone remodeling might be similar in cancellous and cortical bone, occurring in what has been termed the *basic multicellular unit* (BMU), which comprises the osteoclasts, osteoblasts, and osteocytes within the bone-remodeling cavity. Hauge and colleagues[7] demonstrated that cells in the BMU in both bone compartments are not directly contiguous to the bone marrow but are covered by bone-lining cells that seem to be connected to the bone-lining cells of the quiescent bone surface. In turn, these bone-lining cells on the quiescent bone surface are in communication with osteocytes embedded within the bone matrix.[7] Penetrating the canopy of bone-lining cells and presumably serving as a conduit for the cells needed in the BMU are capillaries.[7] The BMU (consisting of osteoclasts, osteoblasts, and osteocytes) is placed within the bone-remodeling compartment which comprises the BMU, the canopy of bone-lining cells, and the associated capillaries.[7]

Given this structure, it becomes easier to understand the key role that osteocytes have in controlling bone remodeling despite being imprisoned in the bone matrix. It is clear that osteocytes can sense microcracks and mechanical strain and be responsive to changes in the hormonal milieu of the bone (eg, glucocorticoids), essentially triggering bone remodeling, perhaps by communicating with bone-lining cells.[8,9] By analogy with remodeling in cortical bone, which is clearly associated with growth of a blood vessel into the remodeling

[a] Department of Rheumatology and Physical Medicine, Erasme University Hospital, (Hôpital Erasme) Université Libre de Bruxelles, 808 Route de Lennik, 1070 Bruxelles, Belgium
[b] Department of Rheumatology, Centre Hospitalier Universitaire de Liege Sart Tilman, 4000 Liège, Belgium
* Corresponding author.
E-mail address: valerie.gangji@erasme.ulb.ac.be (V. Gangji).

Orthop Clin N Am 40 (2009) 213–221
doi:10.1016/j.ocl.2008.10.009

site,[10] the presumed ingrowth of a capillary into the bone-remodeling compartment provides the vascular supply for the cells in the BMU of cancellous bone and might also provide the necessary osteoclasts and, subsequently, the osteoblasts that are needed for bone remodeling in both cancellous and cortical bone. Within the BMU, preosteoblastic cells, which express RANKL,[11] probably control the differentiation of osteoclasts from hematopoietic progenitors. In turn, completion of the bone resorption phase is followed by a wave of bone formation driven, in part, by factors produced by the osteoclast that stimulate osteoblast differentiation and activity, perhaps via direct cell–cell contact between the osteoclast and osteoblast. In the context of this orchestrated activity in the BMU, a number of cells are targeted by the ON disease—the osteoblast, the osteocyte, and possibly the endothelial cell in the capillaries.

OSTEONECROSIS, A BONE DISEASE

Although numerous studies concerning the pathogenesis of ON have been presented, the pathophysiologic mechanisms that may be involved continue to be debated. Different mechanisms leading to ischemia have been postulated, including fat emboli,[12] microvascular tamponade of the blood vessels of the femoral head by marrow fat,[13] retrograde embolization of the marrow fat,[14] and intravascular coagulation.[15] Nevertheless, none of those mechanisms explore the necrotic lesion as a bone disease. In the early 1980s, the concept of accumulative cell stress was advanced, which is a theory that proposes that bone cells are exposed to multiple insults or stresses, the effects of which accumulate to the point that the cells cannot sustain themselves and die.[16] Better understanding of bone biology and the risk factors for ON indicated that those mechanisms should be revisited. Indeed, ON is characterized by apoptosis of the osteocytes and cancellous bone-lining cells in the necrotic lesion but also at a distance of the lesion in the proximal femur.[17] The replicative capacities of osteoblastic cells obtained from the intertrochanteric area of the femur are reduced in ON patients when compared with patients who have osteoarthritis.[4] The number and the activity of fibroblast colony-forming units, reflecting the number of mesenchymal stem cells that could potentially give rise to mature osteoblasts, have been shown to be decreased in ON.[2,3] Moreover, the function of the capillaries serving as a conduit for the cells needed in the BMU and providing blood supply within the bone-remodeling compartment could be altered by emboli or thrombosis.[12,14] This altered bone remodeling can be responsible for three different events in the pathogenesis of ON: (1) the appearance of ON itself, (2) the bone repair that occurs after ON, and (3) its evolution to the subchondral fracture. First, glucocorticoids inhibit osteoblastogenesis and promote osteoblast and osteocyte apoptosis.[18,19] The osteocyte apoptosis could disrupt the mechanosensory role of these cells and prevent the adaptation of bone to ischemia and the medullary changes seen in the early stages of ON.[19–21] The decrease in osteoblast capacity to proliferate could reflect the disruption of the mechanosensory role of the osteocyte canalicular network and explain the evolution from marrow ischemia and edema to ON.[4] Second, at a very early stage, a sufficient repair capability would make the lesion reversible. An insufficient repair mechanism related to a decrease in bone formation might explain the evolution to a further stage of ON and to the subchondral fracture. The rate of bone formation is indeed largely determined by the number of osteoblasts, which, in turn, is determined by the rate of replication of progenitors.[22] Third, the altered capillary function enables the stem cells to travel from the bone marrow to the bone surface to meet the need in bone remodeling necessary to heal the necrotic lesion.

ADULT STEM CELLS

Adult stem cells are capable of maintaining, generating, and replacing terminally differentiated cells within their own specific tissue as a consequence of physiologic cell turnover or tissue damage due to injury.[23] Stem and progenitor cell populations are the upstream components of continuous systems of cell renewal in virtually all human tissues. The most accessible adult stem cells are the hematopoietic ones which primarily reside in the bone marrow but can now be more easily collected in the blood through cytapheresis. The hematopoietic system has traditionally been seen as an organized, hierarchic system with multipotent, self-renewing stem cells at the top, committed progenitor cells in the middle, and lineage-restricted precursor cells which give rise to terminally differentiated cells at the bottom. The bone marrow contains hematopoietic stem cells that give rise to blood cells (red blood cells, leukocytes, and platelets) and that move between bone marrow and peripheral blood, and mesenchymal stem cells.

Mesenchymal stromal cells (MSCs) are nonhematopoietic stromal cells that were first isolated from the bone marrow and subsequently from other adult connective tissues. They exhibit a multilineage differentiation capacity and can develop into diverse cells, including adipocytes, osteoblasts, chondrocytes, myocytes, tenocytes, and neural cells.[24–28] They can contribute to the regeneration of mesenchymal tissues such as bone, cartilage, muscle, ligament, tendon, adipose, and stroma; however, this classic paradigm of stem cell differentiation restricted to its organ-specific lineage is being challenged by the suggestion that adult stem cells, including hematopoietic stem cells, retain a developmental plasticity that allows them to differentiate across boundaries of lineage and tissue.[29,30] Stem cells derived from bone, bone marrow, and peritrabecular tissues in cancellous bone, periosteum, cartilage, muscle, fat, and vascular pericytes are capable of differentiation into multiple phenotypes, including bone, cartilage, tendon, ligament, fat, muscle, and nerve.[31–34] This characteristic has important implications with regard to the design of tissue engineering strategies in that cells derived from one tissue might be useful in forming other tissue types.

Bone marrow aspirates and trabecular bone have both been identified as sources of MSCs, although the quantity obtained from aspirates is less than 0.01%.[35,36] In the laboratory, MSCs from bone marrow can be isolated and expanded using relatively simple protocols based on culture expansion of adherent cells. Expanded MSCs can be guided along specific differentiation pathways in culture by using specific media that contain growth factors or other substances such as dexamethasone (**Fig. 1**).[24,34]

In bone, the continuous remodeling requires the formation of many new osteoblasts. Osteoblasts, in turn, are continuously derived from a much smaller number of preosteoblasts and upstream progenitor cells. The number of true stem cells needed to support this process may be very small (on the average, less than 1 in 20,000 nucleated cells in native marrow).[35] MSCs are thought to be reservoirs of reparative cells, which lack specific tissue characteristics and are ready under different signals to mobilize and differentiate into cells of a connective tissue lineage. The activation of stem cells and the proliferation of progenitor cells to form new osteoblasts are vastly accelerated as a result of trauma, fracture, inflammation, necrosis, and tumors.[37] The mobilization and differentiation of MSCs can be influenced by chemotaxis and interactions with the extracellular matrix through transmembrane proteins such as integrins;[38,39] however, in many cases, MSCs appear to differentiate toward the local cell population under the influence of the microenvironment.

STEM CELLS IN BONE REPAIR

Bone marrow cells contribute to bone repair after systemic or local transplantation in animals and humans. The feasibility of allogeneic bone marrow transplantation to treat a systemic bone disease

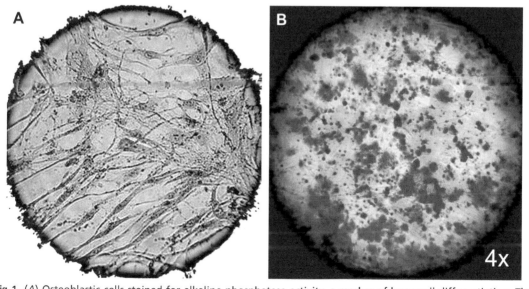

Fig. 1. (*A*) Osteoblastic cells stained for alkaline phosphatase activity, a marker of bone cell differentiation. The osteoblastic cells were obtained from human bone marrow culture in osteogenic media. (*B*) Capacity of the osteoblastic cells to mineralize when cultured in osteogenic media. The osteoblastic cells were obtained from human bone marrow culture in osteogenic media and were allowed to undergo cell differentiation until nodule of mineralization (stained with alizarin red) occurred.

was demonstrated in children with severe osteogenesis imperfecta.[40] In that study, functional marrow-derived mesenchymal cells engrafted and contributed to the formation of new dense bone. The percentage of grafted osteoblasts could not be improved after the transplantation of mesenchymal stem cells only (plastic adherent marrow stromal cells).[41] The interpretation of these observations was that cells other than those in the adherent population, where mesenchymal cells are thought to reside, are potent transplantable progenitors of osteoblasts, consistent with laboratory studies showing that nonadherent cells can give rise to bone. It was demonstrated in the mouse that transplantation of adherent cells would allow an engraftment of transplanted adherent cells representing 1.5% of osteocytes and osteoblasts. Transplantation of nonadherent cells in contrast yielded clusters of donor cells that accounted for 18% of such bone cells. These data showed that the nonadherent marrow cells have a more robust bone repopulating activity than do adherent cells after systemic infusion and that there are two presumably distinct populations of marrow cells with the capacity to generate osteoprogenitors.

For local bone disease, several experimental approaches in animal models have been used to elicit bone formation in segmental bone defects, including implantation of bone marrow,[42] of MSCs,[43] of osteoconductive extracellular matrix scaffolds,[44,45] and of bone morphogenetic proteins (BMPs) in various matrix.[46,47]

In humans, only a few studies have evaluated the efficacy of bone marrow implantation in bone disorders such as nonunion, spinal fusion, or ON (**Table 1**). Goel colleagues[48] evaluated the effect of percutaneous bone marrow grafting in patients with a tibial nonunion, resulting in union in most patients. Siwach colleagues[49] treated 72 patients who had delayed or nonunion of a fracture or poor regeneration in segmental bone transportation or limb lengthening with a percutaneous injection of autologous bone marrow. They achieved union in 68 of 72 patients. Outcomes in these procedures seem to be influenced by the number of MSCs injected into a nonunion. It has been reported that 20 mL of bone marrow is needed to generate 3 mL of new bone.[50,51]

STEM CELLS IN VASCULAR REPAIR

Endothelial progenitor cells have been proposed to circulate in adult organisms and to be recruited and incorporated into sites of physiologic and

Table 1
Evidence to support the therapeutic use of bone marrow transplantation in humans

Reference	Bone Disease	Type of Study	Results
Horwitz and colleagues, 1999[40]	Osteogenesis imperfecta	Prospective study	Mesenchymal cells engrafted and contributed to the formation of new bone
Healey and colleagues, 1990[70]	Nonunion after osteosarcoma resection	Retrospective study	Union in 5/8 patients in 12 weeks
Connolly and c olleagues, 1991[71]	Tibial nonunion	Retrospective study	Union in 18/20 patients
Goel and colleagues, 2005[48]	Tibial nonunion	Prospective study	Union in 15/20 patients in 14 weeks
Siwach and colleagues, 2001[49]	Nonunion of a fracture or poor regeneration in segmental bone transportation or limb lengthening	Retrospective study	Bone union achieved in 68/72 patients
Hernigou and colleagues, 2005[50]	Atrophic nonunion of tibial diaphysis	Retrospective study	Union in 53/60 patients
Gangji and colleagues, 2004[5]	ON of the femoral head	Controlled double-blind study	Delay of ON progression
Hernigou and colleagues, 2002[6]	ON of the femoral head	Prospective study	Delay of ON progression

pathologic neovascularization.[52,53] New therapeutic approaches to promote angiogenesis evolved when it was suggested that the infusion of circulating bone marrow–derived stem or endothelial progenitor cells may improve blood flow recovery in various ischemic models.[52,54] Thus far, one cannot conclude whether these effects can be attributed to the incorporation of stem cells into the wall of new vessels or to cytokines released by chemoattracted bone marrow cells inducing the proliferation of resident endothelial and smooth muscle cells. Recently, Kinnaird colleagues[55] indicated that cultured human bone-derived stromal cells promote arteriogenesis through paracrine mechanisms. They demonstrated that the expression of genes encoding for cytokines related to arteriogenesis (vascular endothelial growth factor [VEGF], fibroblast growth factor-2 [FGF-2], interleukin-6, placental growth factor) was up-regulated. Moreover, in a murine hind limb ischemia model, intramuscular injection of the cultured medium of those bone-derived stromal cells improved collateral blood flow recovery and limb function. It was concluded that paracrine signaling and not cell incorporation may be an important mediator of bone marrow cell therapy in tissue ischemia. Other studies using different approaches had the same conclusions that stem cells promote vasculature growth by their paracrine effects and not by incorporation into the wall of growing vessels.[56,57]

Similarly, a controlled and randomized trial of therapeutic angiogenesis for patients with limb ischemia by autologous transplantation of bone marrow cells explained their therapeutic effect by the injection of endothelial stem cells and by the release of angiogenic factors (VEGF, FGF-2) and angiopoietin-2, which are known to have important functions in maturation and maintenance of the vascular system.[58] Furthermore, in the context of bone disease, Wang colleagues[59] showed that increased VEGF production by osteoblastic cells has a marked anabolic effect on bone, apparently due to increased angiogenesis and subsequent influx of osteoblasts onto bone surface.

The potential of bone marrow mononuclear cell implantation for angiogenesis stimulation has also been demonstrated in patients sustaining myocardial infarction. Infarcted myocardium was reported as repairable by intramyocardial and intracoronary bone marrow cell transplantation.[60–62]

CELLULAR THERAPY IN OSTEONECROSIS OF THE FEMORAL HEAD

Studies on the treatment of ON using cellular therapy from the first report in 1994 to the present are reviewed herein. Autologous bone marrow transplantation was reported for the first time in a patient sustaining ON of the humeral head due to sickle cell anemia. Hernigou colleagues[63,64] reported the case of a 13-year-old patient who had ON of the humeral head secondary to sickle cell disease.[64] The transplantation by marrow intravenous infusion was performed after administration of chemotherapy and total lymphoid irradiation to suppress the immune response. The donor was an HLA-identical sibling who was heterozygous for sickle cell anemia. Three months after the transplantation, radiographs showed rapid reconstruction of the left proximal humerus epiphysis, and T1-weighted MR images demonstrated a tendency toward normalization of the marrow signal in this region. In addition, pain and range of motion considerably improved. Thereafter, Hernigou and colleagues[5,6] and Gangji and colleagues studied the efficacy of bone marrow implantation into the necrotic lesion of ON of the femoral head. A total of 400 mL of bone marrow was aspirated from the anterior iliac crest with the patient under general anesthesia and then transferred into a bone marrow collection kit. The rest of the bone marrow preparation was performed in a sterile room in the cellular and molecular therapy unit. In the mean time, the second step of the procedure, the core decompression, was accomplished. Under fluoroscopic control, a 3-mm trephine was inserted manually through the trochanter, the neck, and the head of the femur to the necrotic lesion. The tip of the trephine was placed at a distance of 2 to 3 mm from the articular cartilage (**Fig. 2**). In the cellular and molecular therapy unit, the bone marrow was filtered to eliminate bone spicules, fat, and cellular debris. Mononuclear cells were then isolated on a cell separator and concentrated to a final volume of 50 mL. This bone marrow was injected through the trephine placed into the necrotic lesion.

Gangji colleagues[5] studied 13 patients (18 hips) with stage I or II (without subchondral fracture) ON of the femoral head according to the system of the Association Research Circulation Osseous in a controlled double-blind trial. The associated risk factors were corticosteroid therapy and alcohol abuse in all but two patients. The hips were allocated to a program of core decompression only (control group) or core decompression and implantation of bone marrow mononuclear cells (bone marrow graft group). The outcomes were safety, clinical symptoms, and disease progression. After 24 months of follow-up, there was a significant reduction in pain and joint symptoms within the bone marrow graft group ($P = .021$). At 24 months, five of the eight hips in the control

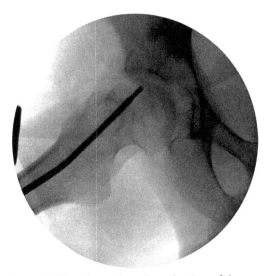

Fig. 2. Profile radiograph made at the time of the core decompression and bone marrow implantation. This 3-mm trephine is introduced by hand under fluoroscopy into the anterosuperior region of the femoral head, and the tip is placed into the necrotic lesion at 3 mm from the subchondral bone.

group had deteriorated to stage III (subchondral fracture), whereas only one of the ten hips in the bone marrow graft group had progressed to this stage ($P = .016$). Survival analysis showed a significant difference in the time to collapse between the two groups. In addition, in the bone marrow graft group, the volume of the necrotic lesion decreased by 35% after 24 months.

Similarly, Hernigou and Beaujean[6] reported the results of a prospective study of 189 hips in 116 patients treated with core decompression and bone marrow grafting in 2002. The patients were followed up from 5 to 11 years with a mean of 7 years. The associated risk factors were corticosteroids for 16% of the hips, alcohol abuse for 30%, sickle cell disease for 34%, organ transplantation for 11%, idiopathic for 5%, and miscellaneous causes for 4%. The outcomes were changes in clinical symptoms, progression in radiographic stages, and the need for hip replacement. When patients were treated before collapse (stage I and II), hip replacement was done in 9 of the 145 hips. Total hip replacement was necessary in 25 hips among the 44 hips operated after collapse (stage III and IV). The number of MSCs implanted was significantly lower in ON attributable to corticosteroid therapy, alcohol abuse, or organ transplantation than in patients with sickle cell disease. The different number of transplanted progenitor cells might have had an influence on the outcome.

Altogether, the two studies showed great improvement in femoral head preservation after stem cell implantation in early stage ON of the femoral head.

HYPOTHESIS FOR THE EFFICACY OF MARROW CELL IMPLANTATION INTO THE OSTEONECROTIC LESION

Recent advances in the understanding of the pathophysiology of ON suggest that a decrease in the mesenchymal stem cell pool of the proximal femur and in the osteoblastic cell proliferation rate might not provide enough osteoblasts to meet the needs of bone remodeling in the early stages of the disease. An insufficiency of osteogenic cells could explain the inadequate repair mechanism that is postulated, leading to femoral head collapse. The effectiveness of bone marrow cells may be related to the availability of stem, mesenchymal, and endothelial stem cells endowed with osteogenic and angiogenic properties, arising from an increase in the supply of such cells to the femoral head via bone marrow implantation. Indeed, in the early stages of ON, creating sufficient repair capacity through the implantation of osteogenic cells could make the lesions reversible. In a study performed by the authors, the volume of the necrotic lesion decreased by 35% in bone marrow–grafted patients, whereas it increased by 23% in the control group. This finding also suggests that necrotic lesions might be reversible. The efficacy of BMPs like BMP-2 or BMP-7 in treating bone diseases such as nonunions[65] or ON[66] could be explained by the same mechanisms, because they have the ability to initiate new bone formation by recruiting mesenchymal stem cells and stimulating their differentiation into osteoprogenitor cells. Another possible explanation for the therapeutic effect of bone marrow implantation is that injected marrow cells supply skeletal and angiogenic factors resulting in increased osteogenesis and angiogenesis.[59] FGF-2,[67,68] transforming growth factor-β,[69] platelet-derived growth factor, and VEGF contained in the bone marrow may also serve as a therapeutic substrate to enhance bone formation. They have indeed demonstrated their ability to increase bone formation in fracture repair[67,69] and ON.[68] Nevertheless, larger trials and the use of other techniques are needed to fully understand the results obtained with cellular therapy in ON, because it is not possible thus far to localize the bone marrow cells after the injection or to demonstrate that the bone repair originated from the injected bone marrow cells.

SUMMARY

Pioneer trials of bone marrow cell implantation in the early stages of ON have shown the safety as well as some degree of clinical efficacy of this new therapeutic approach. This success should modify the treatment of early stage ON in the future. In the meantime, larger controlled and randomized trials aimed at confirming these encouraging results are needed. Improvement in clinical results will only be possible through further optimization of the cellular product, including improved methods of intraoperative bone marrow harvest, concentration, and selection of subpopulations of progenitor cells, along with the improvement of stem cell delivery system and the selection of cellular products adapted to the pathophysiology of bone repair in ON. Human clinical studies are unlikely to be sufficient in identifying the respective role of each of these potential mechanisms of stem cell therapy, highlighting the need for the parallel conduct of laboratory and animal studies. These recent advances in the use of stem cell biology may improve its therapeutic potential.

REFERENCES

1. Lieberman JR, Berry DJ, Mont MA, et al. Osteonecrosis of the hip: management in the 21st century. J Bone Joint Surg Am 2003;52:337–55.

2. Hernigou P, Beaujean F. Abnormalities in the bone marrow of the iliac crest in patients who have osteonecrosis secondary to corticosteroid therapy or alcohol abuse. J Bone Joint Surg Am 1997;79:1047–53.

3. Hernigou P, Beaujean F, Lambotte JC. Decrease in the mesenchymal stem cell pool in the proximal femur in corticosteroid-induced osteonecrosis. J Bone Joint Surg Br 1999;81:349–55.

4. Gangji V, Hauzeur JP, Schoutens A, et al. Abnormalities in the replicative capacity of osteoblastic cells in the proximal femur of patients with osteonecrosis of the femoral head. J Rheumatol 2003;30:348–51.

5. Gangji V, Hauzeur JP, Matos C, et al. Treatment of osteonecrosis of the femoral head with implantation of autologous bone marrow cells: a pilot study. J Bone Joint Surg Am 2004;86-A:1153–60.

6. Hernigou P, Beaujean F. Treatment of osteonecrosis with autologous bone marrow grafting. Clin Orthop 2002;405:14–23.

7. Hauge EM, Qvesel D, Eriksen EF, et al. Cancellous bone remodeling occurs in specialized compartments lined by cells expressing osteoblastic markers. J Bone Miner Res 2001;16:1575–82.

8. Everts V, Delaisse JM, Korper W, et al. The bone lining cell: its role in cleaning Howship's lacunae and initiating bone formation. J Bone Miner Res 2002; 17:77–90.

9. Bonewald LF. Osteocyte messages from a bony tomb. Cell Metab 2007;5:410–1.

10. Parfitt AM. The mechanism of coupling: a role for the vasculature. Bone 2000;26:319–23.

11. Eriksen EF, Eghbali-Fatourechi GZ, Khosla S. Remodeling and vascular spaces in bone. J Bone Miner Res 2007;22:1–6.

12. Jones JP Jr. Fat embolism and osteonecrosis. Orthop Clin North Am 1985;16:595–633.

13. Wang GJ, Sweet DE, Reger SI, et al. Fat cell changes as a mechanism of avascular necrosis of the femoral head in cortisone-treated rabbits. J Bone Joint Surg Am 1977;59:729–35.

14. Simkin PA, Downey DJ. Hypothesis: retrograde embolization of marrow fat may cause osteonecrosis. J Rheumatol 1987;14:870–2.

15. Glueck CJ, Freiberg RA, Fontaine RN, et al. Hypofibrinolysis, thrombophilia, osteonecrosis. Clin Orthop 2001;386:19–33.

16. Fisher DE. The role of fat embolism in the etiology of corticosteroid-induced avascular necrosis: clinical and experimental results. Clin Orthop 1978;130:68–80.

17. Calder JD, Pearse MF, Revell PA. The extent of osteocyte death in the proximal femur of patients with osteonecrosis of the femoral head. J Bone Joint Surg Br 2001;83:419–22.

18. O'Brien CA, Jia D, Plotkin LI, et al. Glucocorticoids act directly on osteoblasts and osteocytes to induce their apoptosis and reduce bone formation and strength. Endocrinology 2004;145:1835–41.

19. Weinstein RS, Jilka RL, Parfitt AM, et al. Inhibition of osteoblastogenesis and promotion of apoptosis of osteoblasts and osteocytes by glucocorticoids: potential mechanisms of their deleterious effects on bone. J Clin Invest 1998;102:274–82.

20. Hauzeur JP, Perlmutter N, Appelboom T, et al. Medullary impairment at early stage of non-traumatic osteonecrosis of the femoral head. Rheumatol Int 1991;11:215–7.

21. Weinstein RS, Nicholas RW, Manolagas SC. Apoptosis of osteocytes in glucocorticoid-induced osteonecrosis of the hip. J Clin Endocrinol Metab 2000; 85:2907–12.

22. Shih MS, Cook MA, Spence CA, et al. Relationship between bone formation rate and osteoblast surface on different subdivisions of the endosteal envelope in aging and osteoporosis. Bone 1993;14:519–21.

23. Slack JM. Stem cells in epithelial tissues. Science 2000;287:1431–3.

24. Jones EA, Kinsey SE, English A, et al. Isolation and characterization of bone marrow multipotential mesenchymal progenitor cells. Arthritis Rheum 2002;46: 3349–60.

25. Orlic D, Kajstura J, Chimenti S, et al. Bone marrow cells regenerate infarcted myocardium. Nature 2001;410:701–5.

26. Schor AM, Canfield AE, Sutton AB, et al. Pericyte differentiation. Clin Orthop Relat Res 1995;313:81–91.

27. De BC, Dell'Accio F, Vandenabeele F, et al. Skeletal muscle repair by adult human mesenchymal stem cells from synovial membrane. J Cell Biol 2003; 160:909–18.

28. Black IB, Woodbury D. Adult rat and human bone marrow stromal stem cells differentiate into neurons. Blood Cells Mol Dis 2001;27:632–6.

29. Weissman IL. Stem cells: units of development, units of regeneration, and units in evolution. Cell 2000; 100:157–68.

30. Blau HM, Brazelton TR, Weimann JM. The evolving concept of a stem cell: entity or function? Cell 2001;105:829–41.

31. Connolly J, Guse R, Lippiello L, et al. Development of an osteogenic bone marrow preparation. J Bone Joint Surg Am 1989;71:684–91.

32. Muschler GF, Boehm C, Easley K. Aspiration to obtain osteoblast progenitor cells from human bone marrow: the influence of aspiration volume. J Bone Joint Surg Am 1997;79:1699–709.

33. Patterson TE, Kumagai K, Griffith L, et al. Cellular strategies for enhancement of fracture repair. J Bone Joint Surg Am 2008;90(Suppl 1):111–9.

34. Pittenger MF, Mackay AM, Beck SC, et al. Multilineage potential of adult human mesenchymal stem cells. Science 1999;284:143–7.

35. Connolly JF. Injectable bone marrow preparations to stimulate osteogenic repair. Clin Orthop Relat Res 1995;313:8–18.

36. Tuli R, Seghatoleslami MR, Tuli S, et al. A simple, high-yield method for obtaining multipotential mesenchymal progenitor cells from trabecular bone. Mol Biotechnol 2003;23:37–49.

37. Muschler GF, Midura RJ, Nakamoto C. Practical modeling concepts for connective tissue stem cell and progenitor compartment kinetics. J Biomed Biotechnol 2003;2003:170–93.

38. Metheny-Barlow LJ, Tian S, Hayes AJ, et al. Direct chemotactic action of angiopoietin-1 on mesenchymal cells in the presence of VEGF. Microvasc Res 2004;68:221–30.

39. Pountos I, Jones E, Tzioupis C, et al. Growing bone and cartilage: the role of mesenchymal stem cells. J Bone Joint Surg Br 2006;88:421–6.

40. Horwitz EM, Prockop DJ, Fitzpatrick LA, et al. Transplantability and therapeutic effects of bone marrow–derived mesenchymal cells in children with osteogenesis imperfecta. Nat Med 1999;5: 309–13.

41. Horwitz EM, Gordon PL, Koo WK, et al. Isolated allogeneic bone marrow–derived mesenchymal cells engraft and stimulate growth in children with osteogenesis imperfecta: implications for cell therapy of bone. Proc Natl Acad Sci U S A 2002;99:8932–7.

42. Grundel RE, Chapman MW, Yee T, et al. Autogeneic bone marrow and porous biphasic calcium phosphate ceramic for segmental bone defects in the canine ulna. Clin Orthop Relat Res 1991;266:244–58.

43. Bruder SP, Kraus KH, Goldberg VM, et al. The effect of implants loaded with autologous mesenchymal stem cells on the healing of canine segmental bone defects. J Bone Joint Surg Am 1998;80:985–96.

44. Hollinger JO, Brekke J, Gruskin E, et al. Role of bone substitutes. Clin Orthop Relat Res 1996;324:55–65.

45. Johnson KD, Frierson KE, Keller TS, et al. Porous ceramics as bone graft substitutes in long bone defects: a biomechanical, histological, and radiographic analysis. J Orthop Res 1996;14:351–69.

46. Cook SD, Baffes GC, Wolfe MW, et al. Recombinant human bone morphogenetic protein-7 induces healing in a canine long-bone segmental defect model. Clin Orthop Relat Res 1994;301:302–12.

47. Gerhart TN, Kirker-Head CA, Kriz MJ, et al. Healing segmental femoral defects in sheep using recombinant human bone morphogenetic protein. Clin Orthop Relat Res 1993;293:317–26.

48. Goel A, Sangwan SS, Siwach RC, et al. Percutaneous bone marrow grafting for the treatment of tibial non-union. Injury 2005;36:203–6.

49. Siwach RC, Sangwan SS, Singh R, et al. Role of percutaneous bone marrow grafting in delayed unions, non-unions and poor regenerates. Indian J Med Sci 2001;55:326–36.

50. Hernigou P, Poignard A, Beaujean F, et al. Percutaneous autologous bone marrow grafting for nonunions: influence of the number and concentration of progenitor cells. J Bone Joint Surg Am 2005;87:1430–7.

51. Hernigou P, Poignard A, Manicom O, et al. The use of percutaneous autologous bone marrow transplantation in nonunion and avascular necrosis of bone. J Bone Joint Surg Br 2005;87:896–902.

52. Asahara T, Murohara T, Sullivan A, et al. Isolation of putative progenitor endothelial cells for angiogenesis. Science 1997;275:964–7.

53. Shi Q, Rafii S, Wu MH, et al. Evidence for circulating bone marrow–derived endothelial cells. Blood 1998; 92:362–7.

54. Kocher AA, Schuster MD, Szabolcs MJ, et al. Neovascularization of ischemic myocardium by human bone marrow–derived angioblasts prevents cardiomyocyte apoptosis, reduces remodeling and improves cardiac function. Nat Med 2001;7:430–6.

55. Kinnaird T, Stabile E, Burnett MS, et al. Marrow-derived stromal cells express genes encoding a broad spectrum of arteriogenic cytokines and promote in vitro and in vivo arteriogenesis through paracrine mechanisms. Circ Res 2004;94:678–85.

56. Rehman J, Li J, Orschell CM, et al. Peripheral blood "endothelial progenitor cells" are derived from monocyte/macrophages and secrete angiogenic growth factors. Circulation 2003;107:1164–9.

57. Ziegelhoeffer T, Fernandez B, Kostin S, et al. Bone marrow–derived cells do not incorporate into the adult growing vasculature. Circ Res 2004;94:230–8.

58. Shyu KG, Manor O, Magner M, et al. Direct intramuscular injection of plasmid DNA encoding angiopoietin-1 but not angiopoietin-2 augments revascularization in the rabbit ischemic hindlimb. Circulation 1998;98:2081–7.

59. Wang Y, Wan C, Deng L, et al. The hypoxia-inducible factor alpha pathway couples angiogenesis to osteogenesis during skeletal development. J Clin Invest 2007;117:1616–26.

60. Stamm C, Westphal B, Kleine HD, et al. Autologous bone marrow stem cell transplantation for myocardial regeneration. Lancet 2003;361:45–6.

61. Strauer BE, Brehm M, Zeus T, et al. Repair of infarcted myocardium by autologous intracoronary mononuclear bone marrow cell transplantation in humans. Circulation 2002;106:1913–8.

62. Tse HF, Kwong YL, Chan JK, et al. Angiogenesis in ischaemic myocardium by intramyocardial autologous bone marrow mononuclear cell implantation. Lancet 2003;361:47–9.

63. Hernigou P, Bernaudin F. [Course of bone tissue after bone marrow allograft in adolescents with sickle cell disease]. Rev Chir Orthop Reparatrice Appar Mot 1994;80:138–43.

64. Hernigou P, Bernaudin F, Reinert P, et al. Bone marrow transplantation in sickle cell disease. Effect on osteonecrosis: a case report with a four-year follow-up. J Bone Joint Surg Am 1997;79:1726–30.

65. Johnson EE, Urist MR. Human bone morphogenetic protein allografting for reconstruction of femoral nonunion. Clin Orthop Relat Res 2000;371: 61–74.

66. Lieberman JR, Conduah A, Urist MR. Treatment of osteonecrosis of the femoral head with core decompression and human bone morphogenetic protein. Clin Orthop Relat Res 2004;429:139–45.

67. Radomsky ML, Thompson AY, Spiro RC, et al. Potential role of fibroblast growth factor in enhancement of fracture healing. Clin Orthop Relat Res 1998;355: S283–93.

68. Yang C, Yang SH, Du JY, et al. Basic fibroblast growth factor gene transfection to enhance the repair of avascular necrosis of the femoral head. Chin Med Sci J 2004;19:111–5.

69. Bostrom MP, Asnis P. Transforming growth factor beta in fracture repair. Clin Orthop Relat Res 1998; 355:S124–31.

70. Healey JH, Zimmerman PA, McDonnell JM, et al. Percutaneous bone marrow grafting of delayed union and nonunion in cancer patients. Clin Orthop Relat Res 1990;256:280–5.

71. Connolly JF, Guse R, Tiedeman J, et al. Autologous marrow injection as a substitute for operative grafting of tibial nonunions. Clin Orthop Relat Res 1991; 366:259–70.

Bisphosphonates and Osteonecrosis: Potential Treatment or Serious Complication?

Robin N. Goytia, MD[a], Andrew Salama, DDS, MD[b],
Harpal S. Khanuja, MD[a],*

KEYWORDS

- Osteonecrosis • Bisphosphonates
- Osteonecrosis of the jaw • Avascular necrosis
- Osteonecrosis of the femoral head • BRONJ

The bisphosphonate family of drugs is widely used in clinical practice for the treatment of postmenopausal osteoporosis, Paget's disease of bone, and cancer-related conditions, including bone metastases, and hypercalcemia of malignancy. Oral bisphosphonates are primarily used in the management of osteoporosis, whereas intravenous (IV) forms are most commonly used for malignancy-related conditions. Bisphosphonates have proven efficacious for the treatment of osteoporosis and are approved for prevention of fractures in postmenopausal women.[1] Postmenopausal women with reduced bone density are the greatest at-risk population likely to benefit from bisphosphonate therapy. Approximately 190 million prescriptions for oral bisphosphonate have been dispensed worldwide.[2] The clinical benefits of bisphosphonates stem from a net decrease in bone turnover as a result of the inhibition of the normal resorptive process of bone.

Bisphosphonates are the most clinically important class of antiresorptive agents available. Their potential to treat other diseases characterized by osteoclast-mediated bone resorption has gained attention. This article reviews the use of bisphosphonates to treat osteonecrosis of the femoral head. Bisphosphonates do have side effects, including the paradoxical association with osteonecrosis of the jaw, which is also discussed in detail in this article.

STRUCTURE

Pyrophosphates are circulating inhibitors of bone mineralization. Their three-dimensional structure gives them a high affinity for the calcium ions in bone, but the P-O-P bonds are easily degraded by alkaline phosphatase within the lining osteoclastic cells. Genetic defects in alkaline phosphatase result in osteomalacia because the pyrophosphate attaches to bone and prevents its mineralization. Bisphosphonates are a class of synthetic compounds that are structurally related to pyrophosphates. They have a similar backbone to the pyrophosphates, with the P-O-P bond replaced by a P-C-P bond (**Fig. 1**). This chemical variation allows for a similar three-dimensional structure to pyrophosphate, which gives these compounds a high affinity for bone. Bisphosphonates work by strongly inhibiting bone resorption. Their long metabolic availability is caused by the fact that there is no known enzyme capable of breaking down the P-C-P bond. All drugs within this class share the same backbone but differ in their side chains R1 and R2 (see **Fig. 1**). The different potencies of the bisphosphonates depend on the variations in the molecular structure of these side chains (**Table 1**), which can be divided into nitrogen-containing and non–nitrogen-containing compounds.

[a] Johns Hopkins Orthopaedics at Good Samaritan Hospital, 5601 Loch Raven Boulevard, Professional Office Building, Suite G-1, Baltimore, MD 21239, USA
[b] Blood and Marrow Transplantation Program, University of Maryland Greenebaum Cancer Center, Baltimore, MD, USA
* Corresponding author.
E-mail address: hkhanuj1@jhmi.edu (H.S. Khanuja).

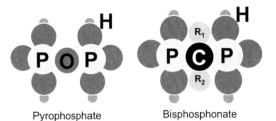

Fig. 1. Three-dimensional structure of pyrophosphates and bisphosphonates. The oxygen is substituted with carbon that makes it resistant to enzymatic breakdown.

MECHANISM OF ACTION

There is no general consensus about which mechanism of action is predominant in vivo, and the mechanisms may be slightly different for each bisphosphonate. Recent work has shown the importance of the chemical structure[3] and whether the side chain contains nitrogen. The non–nitrogen-containing compounds are metabolized into ATP analogues, which then bind to exposed minerals in bone and are absorbed by osteoclasts when bone is resorbed. The ATP analogues become cytotoxic as they accumulate, which leads to decreased cell function and eventually to apoptosis.

The newer generations of bisphosphonates are the nitrogen-containing compounds. The side chains contain a nitrogen amino group and have an increased potency. They work by inhibiting the enzyme farnesyl diphosphate synthase, which normally allows for the formation of two metabolites, farnesyl and geranylgeranyl, which are essential for protein prenylation in the mevalonate pathway (**Fig. 2**). Protein prenylation allows binding of small proteins to the cell membrane. By inhibiting this process, osteoclasts lose cell regulation and

signaling. They exhibit disruption of their ruffled border and apoptosis.[4–6] The mevalonate pathway is the same pathway that is targeted by some classes of cholesterol-lowering drugs.

Although other cell types that use the mevalonate pathway may be affected by bisphosphonates, osteoclasts are the primary cells that mediate their therapeutic effects. This is because bisphosphonates bound to bone are released during resorption and osteoclasts are most directly exposed to them.[3] Bisphosphonates also act on osteoblasts to either increase inhibitors or decrease promoters of osteoclast action or recruitment.

PHYSIOLOGIC EFFECTS

Bisphosphonates have been shown to decrease bone resorption and—to a lesser extent—bone formation, which allows for increased mineralization density and a slight increase in bone volume. There is increased bone strength in the first 5 years and a decreased fracture rate when compared to placebo.[7] The half-life in bone is longer than 10 years, and its long-term effects on bone are unknown. Bisphosphonates have been studied extensively in patients with osteoporosis. Alendronate in doses of 70 mg a week demonstrated increased bone mineral density of the hip, spine, and femur and 50% reduction in fracture risk.[8] Patients demonstrated reduction in bone turnover, as measured by markers for bone resorption and formation.[9] After 10 years of alendronate therapy, there was a significant increase in bone density of the lumbar spine and other sites, and the protective effects against fracture were not diminished.[10] Discontinuation of the drug resulted in a reduction in the protective effects as measured by a reduction in bone mineral density and an increase in markers of bone turnover.[11]

Table 1
Relative potency of bisphosphonates

	Antiresorptive Potency	
	Drug	Relative Potency
Non–N-containing bisphosphonates	Etidronate (Didronel)	1
	Clodronate (Bonefos, Loron)	10
	Tiludronate (Skelid)	0.8
Nitrogenous N-containing bisphosphonates	Pamidronate (APD, Aredia)	20
	Neridronate	100
	Alendronate (Fosamax)	150
	Ibandronate (Boniva)	1000
	Risedronate (Actonel)	2000
	Zoledronate (Zometa)	10,000

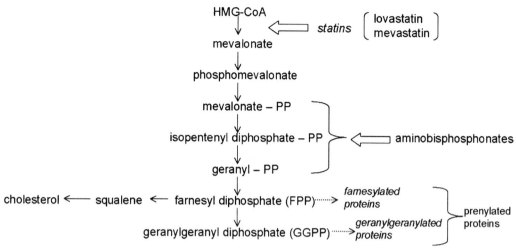

Fig. 2. The Mevalonate pathway (HMG Co A reductase). (*From* Morris CD, Einhorn TA. Bisphosphonates in orthopaedic surgery. J Bone Joint Surg 1005;87A:1609–18; with permission.)

Bisphosphonates are effective in the treatment of Paget's disease. Studies indicate sustained remission and decrease in the level of alkaline phosphatase.[12-14] The antiosteoclast activity of bisphosphonates has also been incorporated as a treatment of skeletal metastatic disease. Not only is osteoclastic activity affected but they also may affect factors that stimulate local tumor growth.[15] Bisphosphonates, particularly zolendonronate, have proven to be highly effective in the treatment of hypercalcemia of malignancy.[16]

There are seven US Food and Drug Administration–approved bisphosphonates: alendronate (Fosamax, Fosamax Plus D), etidronate (Didronel), ibandronate (Boniva), pamidronate (Aredia), risedronate (Actonel, Actonel W/Calcium), tiludronate (Skelid), and zoledronic acid (Reclast, Zometa). They are used primarily to increase bone mass and reduce the risk of fracture in patients with osteoporosis. Bisphosphonates are also used clinically to slow bone turnover in patients with Paget's disease of the bone and treat bone metastases and lower elevated levels of blood calcium in patients with cancer (multiple myeloma, hypercalcemia of malignancy). Off-label use is being studied for other applications, especially diseases in which osteoclastic activity plays an important role (**Box 1**).

Contraindications include women who are pregnant or planning to become pregnant, patients with chronic kidney disease, patients suffering from osteomalacia, and patients with low serum calcium or vitamin D deficiency. In patients with heart failure, coronary artery disease, or diabetes, care needs to be taken because of the high risk of serious adverse effects from atrial fibrillation.[17]

Finally, oral bisphosphonates should not be used in patients with esophageal disease or patients on bed rest who cannot stay upright for an hour.

SIDE EFFECTS

The side effects of bisphosphonates are more severe with use of IV forms (**Fig. 3**). Common side effects from oral bisphosphonates included upper gastrointestinal irritation and esophageal ulceration. Hypercalcemia, hyperparathyroidism, skin rash, and atrial fibrillation are seen with IV and oral forms. There is a concern that the continued use of bisphosphonates over the long-term may result in inhibition of the normal physiologic reparative process of bone. As a result,

---

Box 1
Other uses for bisphosphonates

Pediatric conditions

    Osteogenesis imperfecta

    Fibrous dysplasia

    Legg-Calvé-Perthes

Adult conditions

    Osteoporosis

    Paget's disease of bone

    Metastatic disease of bone

    Arthroplasty

    Fractures and bone healing

    Osteonecrosis

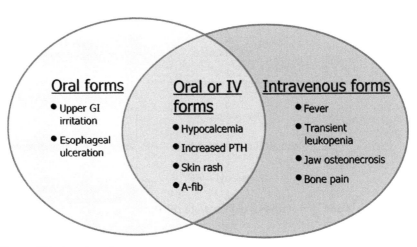

Fig. 3. Side effects of bisphosphonates.

microfractures may accumulate and lead to decreased mechanical properties of bone.[18] There is increasing evidence of an association between the long-term use of bisphosphonates and diaphyseal fractures of the femur.[19] Osteonecrosis of the jaw or jaws is a rare complication of bisphosphonate use. It is seen more commonly with IV forms. This association is discussed in further detail later in this article.

BISPHOSPHONATES AS A TREATMENT OF OSTEONECROSIS OF THE FEMORAL HEAD

Osteonecrosis of the femoral head is the most common diagnosis leading to total hip arthroplasty in young patients. It is a disorder of bony metabolism that likely has vascular injury as a final pathway. No clear cause has been found, and it is likely multifactorial.[20] Multiple associations have been identified (**Table 2**). The pathophysiology is described in more detail elsewhere in this issue. Treatment of osteonecrosis has been primarily surgical and is guided by radiographic staging. As this disease process becomes better understood, more attention is being directed toward medical management with goal of preventing disease progression.

Recent studies investigated the use of bisphosphonates in osteonecrosis. It is presumed that attempted repair by revascularization of necrotic bone results in weakened bone and subsequent collapse and loss of the bony architecture.[21] Because bisphosphonates inhibit osteoclastic activity, they could presumably inhibit the resorption of bone that occurs during revascularization.

Astrand and colleagues[22,23] demonstrated the effects of systemic alendronate and zoledronate on grafted bone in a rat model. They found that the bisphosphonates protected the grafted bone from resorption. In untreated animals, as new bone was incorporated into the graft, the tissue below this new bone formation was resorbed and replaced with hematogenous and fatty tissue. These findings were in contrast to findings in the zolendronate-treated group, in which new bone was seen lining the old graft trabeculae. The treated group had a higher percentage of retained graft bone and a higher percentage of new bone formed.

Bisphosphonates have produced encouraging results in animal models of osteonecrosis.[24–26] Little and colleagues[24] investigated an osteonecrosis model in femoral heads of rats. They found that zolendronic acid preserved the femoral head architecture after traumatic osteonecrosis at 6 weeks compared to controls. A study of the use of ibandronate in immature pigs produced similar findings. Kim and colleagues[25] used ibandronate and observed that the trabecular structure of the osseous epiphysis was preserved and that it prevented femoral head collapse at 8 weeks. A blinded placebo-controlled randomized study in canines with induced osteonecrosis showed that animals treated with oral alendronate had increased mineral density of the femoral head when compared to animals treated with placebo.[26] Bowers and colleagues[26] concluded that increasing the amount of bone in the femoral head may forestall its collapse.

To date few human studies have examined the efficacy of bisphosphonates in osteonecrosis. In one study,[27] a total of 60 patients (100 hips with osteonecrosis at multiple stages) were enrolled. The patients were placed on alendronate, 10 mg/d, calcium, and vitamin D and were advised to be non–weight-bearing. Follow-up times varied,

Table 2
Causes of osteonecrosis

Causes of Osteonecrosis		
Definite	**Probable**	
Major trauma fractures	Corticosteroids, high dosages	Blood clotting disorders
Dislocations	Alcohol	Pancreatitis
Caisson disease (deep-sea divers)	Lipid disturbances	Kidney disease
Sickle cell disease	Connective tissue disease	Liver disease
Radiation therapy	—	Lupus
Chemotherapy	—	Smoking
Arterial disease	—	—
Gaucher's disease	—	—

Courtesy of CORE, Johns Hopkins University, Baltimore, MD.

with 14 patients having less than 1 year follow-up. Results showed that 6% of patients needed surgery by 1 year follow-up and 18% of patients needed it by 2 years. Pain, disability, and walking time improved in their patient population, but range of motion decreased. Radiographic deterioration was seen in 15% of patients at 1 year, 28% of patients at 2 years, and 54% of patients at more than 2 years. The authors concluded that clinically, patients improved and bisphosphonates slowed the progression of the disease. They also stated that the results were better than core decompression. They recommended this treatment of Ficat stages I and II and early stage III osteonecrosis. This study had some limitations because no control was available, the size and location of the lesions were not given, and the follow-up period was short. The results were also confounded by the use of non–weight-bearing in the protoool, which may play a role in the natural history of osteonecrosis.

Lai et al[28] studied 40 patients who were randomly divided into two groups, with Steinberg II and III C lesions with more than 30% head involvement. Twenty patients received 70 mg alendronate weekly for 25 weeks, whereas the control group received a placebo. There was a minimum of 24-month follow-up. Their results showed that in the control group, 20 of 25 hips progressed and 17 of 25 hips required surgical intervention. The alendronate group fared much better: only 4 of 29 hips progressed and only 3 of 29 required surgery. None of the lesions improved radiographically. Their conclusions indicated that alendronate seemed to prevent early collapse of the femoral head. The study period was more than 2 years, and longer follow-up is needed to

confirm that this treatment does not just delay the progression of osteonecrosis.

Nishii and colleagues[29] enrolled 36 hips with either no collapse or only a crescent sign. The diagnosis of osteonecrosis was made within the prior 4 years. Those authors performed an MRI assessment and followed the biochemical markers of bone turnover, urinary alkaline phosphatase, and N telopeptide type I collagen. Twenty hips were given 5 mg of oral alendronate daily for 1 year. The control group of 13 hips did not receive alendronate. All patients had clinical and radiographic follow-up at 3, 6, and 12 months. At 12 months in the alendronate group there was a greater decrease in n-telopeptide, a marker of bone resorption, compared to alkaline phosphatase, a marker of bone formation. There was also a lower incidence of collapse and pain. In advanced C1 and C2 lesions only 1 of the 15 treated hips collapsed compared to 6 of the 11 untreated hips. The authors used the Sugano classification, in which a C1 lesion occupies more than the medial two thirds of the femoral head but does not extend laterally to the acetabular edge and a C2 lesion occupies more than the medial two thirds and extends laterally to the acetabular edge. This study had some limitations, including a small sample size with short follow-up, nonrandomization of patients, and no markers obtained in the untreated group.

Ramachandran and colleagues[30] studied 28 adolescent patients with traumatic osteonecrosis of the femoral head. Twenty-two cases were the result of unstable slipped capital femoral epiphyses, 4 resulted from femoral neck fractures, and 2 resulted from traumatic dislocations. Bone scans were used to identify osteonecrosis after trauma as based on published literature in the pediatric population. The group that demonstrated ischemia on bone scan was treated with bisphosphonates and partial weight-bearing. Seventeen patients were treated for osteonecrosis. Ten patients received pamidronate (1 mg/kg initially, which was increased to 1.5 mg/kg) in alternating monthly cycles; 7 patients received zolendronic acid (0.025–0.05 mg/kg at 3-month intervals). The average duration of follow-up was 38.7 months. Their results showed that 14 of 17 patients were completely pain free and 13 of 17 patients had a normal gait. There was no comment by the authors regarding different results between the groups that received different dosages or medications. Follow-up bone scans showed possible signs of revascularization.

The use of bisphosphonates to slow osteoclastic resorption and prevent collapse has theoretical promise. Although smaller studies exist, to date none has addressed the best dosing regimen, duration of treatment, and whether this treatment delays or prevents progression of the disease. The systemic effects of these medications also need to be considered.

OSTEONECROSIS OF THE JAW: A SERIOUS SIDE EFFECT OF BISPHOSPHONATE USE

Osteonecrosis of the jaw or jaws is relatively rare. It has historically been linked to patients who have received therapeutic doses of radiation for the treatment of head and neck cancer. Radiation-induced osteonecrosis, however, is uncommon even among this group of patients, with an incidence rate of only 10% to 15%.[31] The first report of osteonecrosis of the jaws associated with bisphosphonate therapy was published in 2003, shortly after the introduction of zolendroic acid. Since then, a multitude of case series has been published.[32,33] The clinical constellation of painful exposed bone intraorally was correlated to exposure of bisphosphonates. The medical and dental community was quick to publicize bisphosphonate osteonecrosis through retrospective reviews. In 2004, Novartis, the manufacturer of Zometa and Aredia, distributed a postmarketing experience report that briefly detailed the association of bisphosphonates with osteonecrosis of the jaws.

The term "bisphosphonate-related osteonecrosis of the jaws" (BRONJ) has been coined to distinguish this process from other forms of osteonecrosis of the jaw. The working definition stipulates the following criteria: current or previous exposure to bisphosphonates; exposed, necrotic bone in the maxillofacial region that has persisted for more than 8 weeks; and no history of radiotherapy to the jaws.[34] The exact incidence of BRONJ is not known. Most patients in early reports had either multiple myeloma or metastatic breast cancer treated with IV pamidronate or zolendroic acid. It is estimated that nearly 95% of patients diagnosed with BRONJ are cancer patients who have been treated with the more potent nitrogen-substituted IV bisphosphonates. Ruggiero and colleagues[35] were the first to publish a peer-reviewed retrospective analysis of patients with BRONJ. Only 11% of patients were treated with chronic oral bisphosphonates; the rest received IV bisphosphonates. A meta-analysis review estimated the incidence of BRONJ from IV bisphosphonates to range from 0.8% to 12%.[34]

The number of cases has increased since the development of the nitrogen-containing bisphosphonates zolendroic acid and pamidronate, which are two of the most potent drugs currently in use. Bamias and colleagues[36] noted that no cases of BRONJ were reported before their introduction. Both drugs demonstrate not only higher binding affinity but also higher bioavailability, especially when compared to oral forms.[37] The incidence of BRONJ is reported to be 10% and 4% for zoledronic acid and pamidronate, respectively.[38]

The risk of developing BRONJ with use of oral bisphosphonates is substantially lower. Approximately 170 cases of BRONJ have been reported worldwide with alendronate, mostly in patients who had taken the drug for several years.[39] The estimated incidence of BRONJ among patients treated with weekly alendronate is 0.01% to 0.04%.[40]

CLINICAL PRESENTATION

The clinical hallmark of BRONJ is exposed bone in the oral cavity with or without symptoms, although pain, loose teeth, and gingival erythema may occur before the onset of overt osteonecrosis. The presentation of BRONJ manifests in two distinct groups: patients subjected to previous dental/oral procedures (eg, dental extractions) or trauma and patients who developed symptoms spontaneously. BRONJ has a propensity to occur in sites where the overlying mucosa is relatively thin or in regions prone to trauma (Fig. 4). Spontaneous exposures of bone are nearly twice as likely to occur in dentate patients. The lingual aspect of the mandible is the most common site. Advanced disease within the maxilla may present with chronic sinusitis occasionally accompanied by an oral antral fistula.

Areas of exposed bone are typically small when recognized by patients (<2 cm). Approximately one third of patients present with asymptomatic

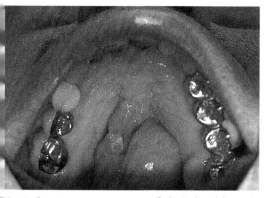

Fig. 4. Spontaneous exposure of devitalized bone in a pre-existing maxillary torus.

exposed bone discovered during a routine dental examination or self-examination.[41] Portions of affected bone may shed spontaneously, occasionally in large segments that contain several teeth. Local factors that contribute to the development of BRONJ include dentoalveolar surgery (eg, dental extraction), endosseous implant placement, and periodontal surgery that involves manipulation of the alveolar bone. Within the oral cavity, BRONJ lesions are far more likely to affect the mandible than the maxilla.

STAGING

A BRONJ staging system has been developed and stratifies patients by symptoms according to the presence of exposed bone, pain, extent of osteolysis within the jaw, presence of inflammation, and evolution of severe infections and pathologic fractures (**Table 3**). Radiographically, the hallmarks of BRONJ include sclerosis, sequestration, and fragmentation (**Fig. 5**). CT seems to be more sensitive

than plain radiography not only in detection of but also delineation of affected bone. MRI has produced poor results when identifying sites of affected bone within the maxillofacial skeleton.[42] The typical radiographic signs may be absent in early stage disease; patients even may have normal-appearing panoramic radiographs.

ETIOLOGY

The etiopathogenesis of BRONJ has not been elucidated. Although the benefits of bisphosphonates outweigh the risks for most patients, attempts have been made to identify patients at higher levels of risk before initiation of therapy. Badros and colleagues[43] reviewed clinical risk factors for the development of BRONJ in patients who had multiple myeloma. The most significant factors related to the development of BRONJ were dental extraction ($P<.009$) and sequential therapy with pamidronate and zolendroic acid ($P<.009$). In another study, sequential therapy was shown to increase cumulative incidence of BRONJ at 5 years among patients who had breast cancer and multiple myeloma.[44]

The relationship between manipulation of the dentoalveolar structures and BRONJ is unclear; however, patients exposed to IV bisphosphonates who have dentoalveolar surgery are at least seven times more likely to develop BRONJ than patients who do not have the surgery.[34] The development of BRONJ also may be a function of time; with each passing year the risk of developing BRONJ increases 57%.[43] Age alone has not been shown to be a contributing factor. The incidence among children receiving IV bisphosphonates has not been demonstrated.[45] No significant associations with regard to gender, steroids, thalidomide, or stage of malignancy have been noted.[43]

Table 3 Staging of bisphosphonate-related osteonecrosis of the jaws	
BRONJ Staging	**Physical Findings**
At-risk patients	No apparent exposed or necrotic bone in patients who have been treated with either oral or IV bisphosphonates
Stage I	Exposed/necrotic bone in patients who are asymptomatic and have no evidence of infection
Stage II	Exposed/necrotic bone associated with infection as evidenced by pain and erythema in the region of exposed bone with or without purulence
Stage III	Exposed/necrotic bone in patients with pain, infection, and one or more of the following: pathologic fracture, extraoral fistula, or osteolysis extending to the inferior border of the mandible

Adapted from American Association of Oral and Maxillofacial Surgeons. Position paper on bisphosphonate-related osteonecrosis of the jaws. J Oral Maxillofac Surg 2007;65(3):369–76; with permission.

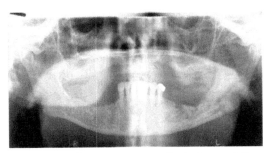

Fig. 5. An orthopantomogram illustrates a 1.5-cm sequestrum. Sclerosis is present along the inferior border of the left mandible. The inferior alveolar canal is obscured by sclerosis.

The total dose of bisphosphonates and the duration of therapy influence the development of BRONJ. Risk increases with drug dose and potency. Zolendroic acid imparted a 30-fold increase in risk, whereas the risk for pamidronate was increased 3.8-fold in one study.[46] The cumulative exposure time to the development of BRONJ varies. Raje and colleagues[42] showed a mean time to diagnosis after treatment initiation of 38.7 months; Kaplan-Meier estimates of time to BRONJ in patients who had multiple myeloma was 8.37 years.[43] The mean duration of drug expose to bone symptoms was significantly less in the study by Marx and colleagues:[41] 14.3 months for pamidronate, 9.4 months for zolendroic acid, and 12.1 months for sequential therapy.

It is unclear whether medical comorbidities play a causal role in BRONJ. Patients with pre-existing reduced bone density are at greater risk. Risk is also increased for patients diagnosed with multiple myeloma compared to patients who have metastatic breast cancer.[44] Among patients without cancer, the most common risk factor has been dental procedures, which was present in nearly 90% of patients.[47] Obesity and smoking also have been linked to the development of BRONJ.[45] Poor oral hygiene and periodontal disease are associated with a sevenfold increase in risk.[44]

Several mechanisms for BRONJ have been suggested; however, the scientific data to substantiate these proposed theories are weak. As systemically administered drugs, bisphosphonates theoretically bind to bone throughout the skeleton, but the jaws are disproportionately affected by side effects. Bone turnover in the tooth-bearing regions of the jaws is relatively high as a function of daily bone remodeling around the teeth and the physiologic stresses of mastication.[48] Bisphosphonate-mediated osteoclast inhibition limits bone remodeling and mitigates new bone growth. A net decrease in bone remodeling is thought to limit the growth of new capillaries, and osteonecrosis ensues. Inadvertent trauma to thin overlying mucosa exposes avascular bone to normal oral bacterial flora, and osteonecrosis ensues.[39]

Bisphosphonates have been found to possess antiangiogenic properties, which may play a role in their antitumor activity.[49] Ferretti and colleagues[50] suggested that the formation of new capillaries is decreased by the inhibition of vascular endothelial growth factor as a result of antiangiogenic properties of bisphosphonates. These properties may play a role in the development of osteonecrosis of the jaws.

TREATMENT OF BISPHOSPHONATE-RELATED OSTEONECROSIS OF THE JAWS

To date, evidence-based guidelines for the management of BRONJ have not been established. Initial attempts to treat exposed bone in the oral cavity with debridement and sequestrectomy were met with unpredictable results. Attempts to cover exposed bone with local tissue flaps after debridement were sometimes counterproductive, and some patients developed subsequent pathologic fractures.[33] Smaller series related promising results with surgical therapy among selected patients.[51]

The American Association of Oral and Maxillofacial Surgeons task force has outlined treatment based on stage of disease with an emphasis on prevention. Before initiating therapy with IV bisphosphonates, patients should undergo a comprehensive dental examination. Elective procedures and simple restorative dentistry should be performed before the beginning therapy. At-risk patients without symptoms or signs require no treatment. Maintenance of good oral hygiene and avoidance of invasive dental procedures are the key components in managing susceptible patients. Early stage disease, in which there is painless exposed bone without infection (stage I), does not benefit from surgical therapy. Antimicrobial mouth rinses and frequent follow-up are recommended. As the disease progresses, patients with painful exposed bone and signs of infection (stage II) may benefit from the inclusion of systemic antibiotics in addition to antimicrobial mouth rinses. Seventy-five percent of patients were stabilized with this regimen in one study.[35] Refractory cases may be treated with long-term IV antibiotics or low-dose suppressive oral penicillins.[34]

Patients in stage III are most likely to benefit from surgery. The extraction of loose teeth should be performed in affected regions of the jaw. Coverage of remaining exposed bone after

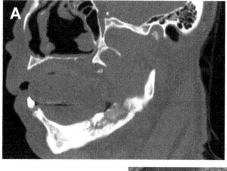
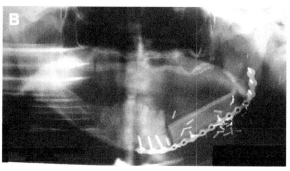
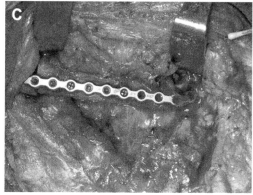

Fig. 6. (A) CT scan (sagittal reconstruction) of the left hemi-mandible demonstrates extensive BRONJ extending to the inferior border of the mandible. (B) Postoperative orthopantomogram of the reconstructed left hemi-mandible. (C) Surgical exposure of the left hemi-mandible after segmental resection and inset of vascularized free fibula flap.

surgical debridement should be attempted with local soft tissue flaps. This is in addition to oral antibiotics and antimicrobial mouth rinses. Complicated stage III disease that involves a pathologic fracture of the mandible or an oral antral communication of the maxilla requires reconstruction. This procedure is accomplished with plates and grafting; however, consolidation of bone grafts in these regions appears less predictable than in patients who do not have BRONJ. Defects involving oral mucosa and bone are aptly treated with osteocutaneous free flaps (osteocutaneous free fibula, deep circumflex iliac artery free flap) (**Fig. 6**). An aggressive surgical approach has been advocated, and promising results have been seen in the small number of patients who actually reach this stage of disease.[52]

The temporary discontinuation of bisphosphonates (drug holidays) in patients with BRONJ is advocated in some clinical situations. There seems to be a limited short-term benefit to stopping bisphosphonates after diagnosis of early stage disease. There is little certainty that stopping bisphosphonates adversely affects the progression or development of new BRONJ lesions.[32] Because the half-life of bisphosphonate is so long, there is no absolute reason to discontinue therapy.[48] A multicenter retrospective review illustrated that patients suffered more skeletal-related events after drug holidays and developed additional or progressive disease when therapy was reinitiated (A.Z. Badros, MD, ChB, personal communication, 2008).

SUMMARY

Oral use of bisphosphonates for osteonecrosis of the hip has shown some early promising results, but most studies contain small sample sizes and relatively short follow-up. The exact mechanism has not been elucidated. We are still in the early stages of understanding how these powerful drugs work, and uncertainty exists regarding dosing and long-term effects. Theoretically, bisphosphonates target the collapse that results from resorption of the necrotic bone in osteonecrosis of the femoral head; however, these systemic drugs have their effects throughout the skeletal system. The consequences of impaired physiologic remodeling have yet to be defined. Long-term use of these drugs needs to be weighed against the possible systemic side effects. Although theoretically their role shows potential, they should be used cautiously and not indefinitely. It is also concerning that although this family of drugs is targeted to treat osteonecrosis of the femoral head, there is an association with its production of osteonecrosis in the jaw.

BRONJ is a relatively new clinical phenomenon associated with exposure to all bisphosphonates, although it occurs far more commonly with the potent IV amino-substituted drugs. The incidence seems to be low with the use of orally administered drugs, whereas the incidence in patients being treated for malignancy is upwards of 10%. All previous studies but one used lower doses of the less potent oral bisphosphonates to successfully treat osteonecrosis of the femoral head. Future research endeavors should help delineate the actual incidence BRONJ. Definitive risk factors have been identified, but the exact developmental mechanism of BRONJ is still under investigation. Most patients seem to have disease limited to early stages, for which surgical therapy is unproven. Currently, the benefits of bisphosphonates outweigh the risks for most patients who have cancer. Nonsurgical treatment modalities have been shown to be effective for stage I and II patients. It is hoped that data from clinical and basic science research will disclose a better comprehension of BRONJ and lead to early diagnosis and improved clinical management.

ACKNOWLEDGMENTS

Special thanks to Dr. Maria Goddard for her assistance in preparation of the manuscript.

REFERENCES

1. Cole Z, Dennison E, Cooper C. Update on the treatment of post-menopausal osteoporosis. Br Med Bull 2008;86:129–43 [epub 2008 May 12].
2. Health, IMS. (2006). "National Prescription Audit Plus™."
3. Morris CD, Einhorn TA. Bisphosphonates in orthopaedic surgery [review]. J Bone Joint Surg Am 2005;87(7):1609–18.
4. Luckman SP, Hughes DE, Coxon FP, et al. Nitrogen-containing bisphosphonates inhibit the mevalonate pathway and prevent post-translational prenylation of GTP-binding proteins, including Ras. J Bone Miner Res 1998;13:581–9.
5. Zhang D, Udagawa N, Nakamura I, et al. The small GTP-binding protein, rho p21, is involved in bone resorption by regulating cytoskeletal organization in osteoclasts. J Cell Sci 1995;108:2285–92.
6. Fisher JE, Rogers MJ, Halasy JM, et al. Alendronate mechanism of action: geranylgeraniol, an intermediate in the mevalonate pathway, prevents inhibition of osteoclast formation, bone resorption, and kinase activation in vitro. Proc Natl Acad Sci USA 1999;96: 133–8.
7. Tonino RP, Meunier PJ, Emkey R, et al. Skeletal benefits of alendronate: 7-year treatment of postmenopausal osteoporotic women. J Clin Endocrinol Metab 2000;85(9):3109–15.
8. Black DM, Cummings SR, Karpf DB, et al. Randomised trial of effect of alendronate on risk of fracture in women with existing vertebral fractures. Fracture Intervention Trial Research Group. Lancet 1996; 348:1535–41.
9. Bauer DC, Black DM, Garnero P, et al. Fracture Intervention Trial Study Group. Change in bone turnover and hip, non-spine, and vertebral fracture in alendronate-treated women: the fracture intervention trial. J Bone Miner Res 2004;19:1250–8.
10. Bone HG, Hosking D, Devogelaer JP, et al. Alendronate Phase III Osteoporosis Treatment Study Group. Ten years' experience with alendronate for osteoporosis in postmenopausal women. N Engl J Med 2004;350:1189–99.
11. Rizzoli R, Greenspan SL, Bone G 3rd, et al. Alendronate Once-Weekly Study Group. Two-year results of once-weekly administration of alendronate 70 mg for the treatment of postmenopausal osteoporosis. J Bone Miner Res 2002;17:1988–96.
12. Siris E, Weinstein RS, Altman R, et al. Comparative study of alendronate versus etidronate for the treatment of Paget's disease of bone. J Clin Endocrinol Metab 1996;81:961–7.
13. Siris ES, Chines AA, Altman RD, et al. Risedronate in the treatment of Paget's disease of bone: an open label, multicenter study. J Bone Miner Res 1998; 13:1032–8.
14. McClung MR, Tou CK, Goldstein NH, et al. Tiludronate therapy for Paget's disease of bone. Bone 1995;17(Suppl 5):493S–6S [Erratum appears in Bone 1996;18: 292].
15. Green JR. Antitumor effects of bisphosphonates. Cancer 2003;97(Suppl 3):840–7.
16. Major P, Lortholary A, Hon J, et al. Zoledronic acid is superior to pamidronate in the treatment of hypercalcemia of malignancy: a pooled analysis of two randomized, controlled clinical trials. J Clin Oncol 2001;19:558–67.
17. Heckbert SR, Li G, Cummings SR, et al. Use of alendronate and risk of incident atrial fibrillation in women. Arch Intern Med 2008;168(8):826–31.
18. Mashiba T, Hirano T, Turner CH, et al. Suppressed bone turnover by bisphosphonates increases microdamage accumulation and reduces some biomechanical properties in dog rib. J Bone Miner Res 2000;15:613–20.

19. Neviaser AS, Lane JM, Lenart BA, et al. Low-energy femoral shaft fractures associated with alendronate use. J Orthop Trauma 2008;22(5):346–50.

20. Mont MA, Jones LC, Hungerford DS. Nontraumatic osteonecrosis of the femoral head: ten years later. J Bone Joint Surg Am 2006;88(5):1117–32 [review].

21. Glimcher MJ, Kenzora JE. Nicolas Andry award. The biology of osteonecrosis of the human femoral head and its clinical implications: 1. Tissue biology. Clin Orthop Relat Res 1979;(138):284–309.

22. Tägil M, Aspenberg P, Astrand J. Systemic zoledronate precoating of a bone graft reduces bone resorption during remodeling. Acta Orthop 2006;77(1):23–6.

23. Astrand J, Aspenberg P. Topical, single dose bisphosphonate treatment reduced bone resorption in a rat model for prosthetic loosening. J Orthop Res 2004;22(2):244–9.

24. Little DG, Peat RA, Mcevoy A, et al. Zoledronic acid treatment results in retention of femoral head structure after traumatic osteonecrosis in young Wistar rats. J Bone Miner Res 2003;18:2016–22.

25. Kim H, Randall TS, Bian H, et al. Ibandronate decreases femoral head deformity following ischemic necrosis of the capital femoral epiphysis in immature pigs. Trans Annu Meet Orthop Res Soc 2004;29:151.

26. Bowers JR, Dailiana ZH, McCarthy EF, et al. Drug therapy increases bone density in osteonecrosis of the femoral head in canines. J Surg Orthop Adv 2004;13(4):210–6.

27. Agarwala S, Jain D, Joshi VR, et al. Efficacy of alendronate, a bisphosphonate, in the treatment of AVN of the hip: a prospective open-label study. Rheumatology (Oxford) 2005;44(3):352–9 [epub 2004 Nov 30] [Erratum appears in Rheumatology (Oxford) 2005;44(4):569].

28. Lai KA, Shen WJ, Yang CY, et al. The use of alendronate to prevent early collapse of the femoral head in patients with nontraumatic osteonecrosis: a randomized clinical study. J Bone Joint Surg Am 2005;87(10):2155–9.

29. Nishii T, Sugano N, Miki H, et al. Does alendronate prevent collapse in osteonecrosis of the femoral head? Clin Orthop Relat Res 2006;443:273–9.

30. Ramachandran M, Ward K, Brown RR, et al. Intravenous bisphosphonate therapy for traumatic osteonecrosis of the femoral head in adolescents. J Bone Joint Surg Am 2007;89(8):1727–34.

31. Bedwinek JM, Shukovsky LJ, Fletcher GH, et al. Osteonecrosis in patients treated with definitive radiotherapy for squamous cell carcinomas of the oral cavity and naso- and oropharynx. Radiology 1976; 119(3):665–7.

32. Khosla S, Burr D, Cauley J, et al. Bisphosphonate-associated osteonecrosis of the jaw: report of a task force of the American Society for Bone and Mineral Research. J Bone Miner Res 2007;22(10): 1479–91.

33. Marx RE. Pamidronate (Aredia) and zoledronate (Zometa) induced avascular necrosis of the jaws: a growing epidemic. J Oral Maxillofac Surg 2003; 61(9):1115–7.

34. American Association of Oral and Maxillofacial Surgeons. Position paper on bisphosphonate-related osteonecrosis of the jaws. J Oral Maxillofac Surg 2007;65(3):369–76.

35. Ruggiero SL, Mehrotra B, Rosenberg TJ, et al. Osteonecrosis of the jaws associated with the use of bisphosphonates: a review of 63 cases. J Oral Maxillofac Surg 2004;62(5):527–34.

36. Bamias A, Kastritis E, Bamia C, et al. Osteonecrosis of the jaw in cancer after treatment with bisphosphonates: incidence and risk factors. J Clin Oncol 2005;23(34):8580–7.

37. Ezra A, Golomb G. Administration routes and delivery systems of bisphosphonates for the treatment of bone resorption. Adv Drug Deliv Rev 2000; 42(3):175–95.

38. Durie BG, Katz M, Crowley J, et al. Osteonecrosis of the jaw and bisphosphonates. N Engl J Med 2005; 353(1):99–102 [discussion: 99–102].

39. Sarin J, DeRossi SS, Akintoye SO, et al. Updates on bisphosphonates and potential pathobiology of bisphosphonate-induced jaw osteonecrosis. Oral Dis 2008;14(3):277–85.

40. Mavrokokki T, Cheng A, Stein B, et al. Nature and frequency of bisphosphonate-associated osteonecrosis of the jaws in Australia. J Oral Maxillofac Surg 2007;65(3):415–23.

41. Marx RE, Sawatari Y, Fortin M, et al. Bisphosphonate-induced exposed bone (osteonecrosis/osteopetrosis) of the jaws: risk factors, recognition, prevention, and treatment. J Oral Maxillofac Surg 2005;63(11):1567–75.

42. Raje N, Woo SB, Hande K, et al. Clinical, radiographic, and biochemical characterization of multiple myeloma patients with osteonecrosis of the jaw. Clin Cancer Res 2008;14(8):2387–95.

43. Badros A, Weikel D, Salama A, et al. Osteonecrosis of the jaws in multiple myeloma patients: clinical features and risk factors. J Clin Oncol 2006;24: 945–52.

44. Hoff AO, Toth BB, Altundag K, et al. Frequency and risk factors associated with osteonecrosis of the jaw in cancer patients treated with intravenous bisphosphonates. J Bone Miner Res 2008;23(6): 826–36.

45. Brown JJ, Ramalingam L, Zacharin MR, et al. Bisphosphonate-associated osteonecrosis of the jaw: does it occur in children? Clin Endocrinol (Oxf) 2008;68(6):863–7.

46. Wessel JH, Dodson TB, Zavras AI, et al. Zoledronate, smoking, and obesity are strong risk factors for osteonecrosis of the jaw: a case-control study. J Oral Maxillofac Surg 2008;66(4):625–31.

47. Hess LM, Jeter JM, Benham-Hutchins M, et al. Factors associated with osteonecrosis of the jaw among bisphosphonate users. Am J Med 2008; 121(6):475–83 [e3].

48. Marx RE, Cillo JE Jr, Ulloa JJ, et al. Oral bisphosphonate-induced osteonecrosis: risk factors, prediction of risk using serum CTX testing, prevention, and treatment. J Oral Maxillofac Surg 2007;65(12): 2397–410.

49. Santini D, Vespasiani Gentilucci U, Vincenzi B, et al. The antineoplastic role of bisphosphonates: from basic research to clinical evidence. Ann Oncol 2003;14(10):1468–76.

50. Ferretti G, Fabi A, Carlini P, et al. Zoledronic-acid-induced circulating level modifications of angiogenic factors, metalloproteinases and proinflammatory cytokines in metastatic breast cancer patients. Oncology 2005;69(1):35–43.

51. Diego R, D'Orto O, Pagani D, et al. Bisphosphonate-associated osteonecrosis of the jaws: a therapeutic dilemma. Oral Surg Oral Med Oral Pathol Ora Radiol Endod 2007;103(3):e1–5.

52. Engroff SL, Kim DD. Treating bisphosphonate osteonecrosis of the jaws: is there a role for resection anc vascularized reconstruction? J Oral Maxillofac Surg 2007;65(11):2374–85.

Does Statin Usage Reduce the Risk of Corticosteroid-Related Osteonecrosis in Renal Transplant Population?

Muhammad Ajmal, MD[a], A.J. Matas, MD[b],
Michael Kuskowski, PhD[c], Edward Y. Cheng, MD[d],*

KEYWORDS

- Osteonecrosis • Statins • Avascular necrosis
- Transplant • Incidence

Osteonecrosis (ON) is a disabling disease and its pathogenesis is associated with corticosteroid exposure, ethanol usage, coagulapathies, and lupus erythematosus. It is an important orthopedic complication of corticosteroid immunosuppression after solid organ transplantation, occurring with a frequency of 3% to 41%.[1–3] Abnormalities of lipid metabolism, fat overload, and intraosseous hypertension have been cited frequently as important in the development of ON.[4–6] Previous studies suggest that ON develops in 5% to 11% of organ transplant patients within 1 year after the transplant,[7–9] but it is not possible to predict which patients receiving corticosteroids will develop ON. Aside from minimizing the exposure to corticosteroids or other risk factors, there are no definite measures available to prevent ON.[10–12]

Animal and limited clinical data have suggested that statins may have a protective role against ON. Wang and other investigators[13–18] have shown that corticosteroids cause the marrow pluripotent cells to differentiate into fat cells through downregulation of Cbfa1/Runx2 gene expression and osteocalcin promoter activity, while increasing the expression of adipose-specific genes 422(aP2) and PPARγ2. Statins do the opposite, by decreasing adipogenic and stimulating osteogenic differentiation through suppressing PPARγ2 and increasing Cbfa1/Runx2 expression in bone-marrow mesenchymal cells.

The goal of the present study was to determine if statin usage in renal transplantation patients is associated with a reduction in incidence of ON.

MATERIALS AND METHODS
Study Design

The authors' transplant recipient data is prospectively gathered and maintained in a computer database with the funding provided by the National Institutes of Health (NIH, Bethesda, Maryland). Using this database,[10,20] the authors retrospectively identified 3,399 patients who had a renal transplant between January 1985 and December 2003. This time period was selected to allow a minimum follow-up of 3 years after the transplantation. Entry criteria were patients greater than or equal to 16 years of age, first-time renal

This article has been funded by NIH Grant DK13083 (to A.J.M.) and educational grants by Wright Medical Technology, Inc, Arlington, Tenessee and Biomet Inc, Warsaw, Indiana (to E.Y.C.).

[a] Department of Orthopaedic Surgery, Veterans Affairs Hospital, Nashville, Affiliated with Vanderbilt University, 1310 24th Avenue South, Nashville, TN 37212, USA

[b] Department of Surgery, University of Minnesota, 420 Delaware Street SE, Minneapolis, MN 55455, USA

[c] Minneapolis Veteran's Affairs Medical Center, 1 Veterans Drive, Minneapolis, MN 55417, USA

[d] Department of Orthopaedic Surgery, University of Minnesota, 2512 South 7th Street, Suite 200, Minneapolis, MN 55454, USA

* Corresponding author.

E-mail address: cheng002@umn.edu (E.Y. Cheng).

orthopedic.theclinics.com

transplants, and with no prior corticosteroid exposure. Statin usage was defined as being on a statin drug at the time of transplant or initiated within 31 days after transplant, and continuing for at least 1-year duration. This time period was selected based upon the finding that ON commonly develops within the first year after transplantation.[7–9] The indication for statin treatment was hypercholesterolemia. Dosages were adjusted by the treating physician until the cholesterol level was reduced to the clinically appropriate target range. The most commonly used statin drugs were Advicor (500-mg niacin + 20-mg lovastatin; Kos Pharmaceuticals, Inc, Cranbury, New Jersey), atorvastatin (Lipitor, Pfizer Inc., New York, New York), crivastatin (Baycol, Bayer AG, Leverkusen, Germany), rosuvastatin (Crestor, AstraZeneca PLC, London, UK), fluvastatin (Lescol, Novartis AG, Basel, Switzerland), lovastatin (Mevacor, Merck and Co., Inc., Whitehouse Station, New York), pravastatin (Pravachol, Bristol-Myers Squibb Co., New York, New York), and simvastatin (Zocor, Merck and Co., Inc.).

Power Analysis

The authors performed a power analysis to determine what potential difference in ON-free survivorship would have been detectable, given the size of the patient cohort, at 5 and 10 years after transplantation. At power equaling 95% and level of significance being $P = .05$, the data were sufficient to detect a difference in ON-free survival, if it was present, of 3% at 5 years (statin exposure group 91% versus nonstatin exposure group 94%) and 5% at 10 years (statin exposure group 88% versus nonstatin exposure group 93%).

Demographics

There were 2,881 patients who met the entry criteria: 1,752 (61%) male and 1,129 (39%) female. Among the 2,881 patients, 1,619 had varying levels of exposure to statins; however, only 338 patients met the authors' on-statins definition.

There were 338 (12%) patients in the statin cohort and 2,543 (88%) in the nonstatin cohort (**Table 1**). In the statin cohort, 180 (53%) were males and 158 (47%) were females. In the nonstatin cohort, 1,572 (62%) were males and 971 (38%) were females. The mean age of the overall patient cohort was 43 years (range, 16–77 years) and mean follow-up was 128 months (range, 36–242 months). In the statin cohort, mean age was 47 years (range, 23–74 years) and mean follow-up was 91 months (range, 43–229 months); in the nonstatin cohort, the mean age was 42 years (range, 16–247 years) and mean follow-up was

Table 1 Demographics of study cohort	
Variable	Value
Total number of patients	2,881
Male: female	1,752 (61%):1,129 (39%)
Age (years)[a]	43 ± 12.8 (16–77)
Follow-up (months)[a]	128 ± 57.8 (36–242)
Statin usage: no statin usage	338/2,881 (12%):2,543/ 2,881 (88%)
Total number of patients with ON	195 (7%)
Total number of sites affected	286
Femoral head	278
Other	8

[a] Values are expressed as mean ± standard deviation, with range in parentheses.

136 months (range, 43–247 months). The most common primary diagnosis that led to end-stage renal failure was diabetic nephropathy. Patients were prospectively followed by regular clinic visits. The authors depended upon self-reporting of fractures, ON, joint pain, or arthritis (not otherwise specified) as noted in the charts. The medical record was reviewed for any patients reporting joint pain (not otherwise specified) to verify the diagnosis and look for other possible etiologies. Data gathered consisted of name, gender, age, indication, and transplant type (living twin, living non-twin, cadaver), transplant date, preemptive transplant (transplant without prior dialysis), post-dialysis transplant, number of rejection episodes, and statin drug usage (yes/no). No patients were contacted specifically for this study and only chart data was reviewed.

Statistical Analysis

Multivariate Cox regression tests[21] were used to analyze ON-free survival on statins and other variables, including gender, rejection episodes, and year of transplantation. Survivorship analysis was performed using Kaplan-Meier methods, with the endpoint defined as occurrence of ON.[22] Log-rank and Wilcoxon tests were performed for comparison of data between the statins versus nonstatin cohort to determine whether there was a relationship between the time course for development of ON and statin usage. The data were analyzed using SAS for Windows statistical software package (Version 9.1 2003; SAS Institute Inc, Cary, North Carolina).

RESULTS

In the overall patient cohort of 2,881 patients, 195 (7%) developed ON in 286 joints. In the femoral head, 96 patients developed ON unilaterally and 91 bilaterally. Eight patients had involvement of other bones. Among the 338 patients in the statin cohort, 15 patients (4.4%) developed ON at 23 sites (all involving the femoral head). In the nonstatin cohort of 2,543 patients, 180 patients (7%) developed ON at 263 sites (255 femoral heads and 8 other sites). ON-free survival stratified by statin usage did not show a relationship between statin exposure and development of ON ($P = .14$, log-rank) (**Fig. 1**). At 5 years, the ON-free survivorship for those patients on statins versus those not on statins was 96% plus or minus 2.1% (95% confidence interval or CI) versus 94% plus or minus 1.0% (95% CI). Cox regression revealed that statin usage did not predict ($P = .8$) ON-free survival. Other variables (**Table 2**) that were associated with a higher incidence of ON were (*i*) male gender ($P = .008$), (*ii*) higher number of rejection episodes ($P = .009$), and (*iii*) earlier year of transplant ($P = .01$).

DISCUSSION

Osteonecrosis is an important orthopedic complication of corticosteroid immunosuppression after solid-organ transplantation with poorly understood pathogenesis. Aside from minimizing the exposure to corticosteroids or other risk factors, there are no definite measures available to prevent ON. The authors' goal was to determine if statin usage in renal transplantation patients is associated with a reduction in incidence of ON.

Prior reports suggest a relationship between statins and ON. Li and colleagues[15] and Wang and colleagues[18] have shown corticosteroids cause the marrow pluripotent cells to differentiate into fat cells through down-regulation of Cbfa1/Runx2 gene expression and osteocalcin promoter activity, while increasing the expression of adipose-specific genes 422(aP2) and PPARγ2. Statins do the opposite by decreasing adipogenic and stimulating osteogenic differentiation through suppressing PPARγ2 and increasing Cbfa1/Runx2 expression in bone-marrow mesenchymal cells.[13,14,16,23] This may or may not be related to their known mechanism of action in lowering cholesterol via inhibition of 3-hydroxy-3-methylglutaryl coenzyme-A reductase. The effect of corticosteroids and statins is concentration- and time-dependent.[13–16,23–26] Corticosteroids are a clear risk factor for ON, and therefore, with these animal and laboratory findings in mind, the authors investigated whether or not statins have a protective role against ON in human beings.

Pritchett's[17] study in 2001 reported a protective role of statins against ON in human beings. He reported the incidence of ON in 1% of 284 patients on statins, which appears less than the historical incidence of 5% to 11% previously reported in the literature.[7–9] Pritchett concluded that statins may protect against the development of ON in patients receiving corticosteroid treatment. However, his study was retrospective, with poorly controlled entry criteria. There were no controls other than historical controls. In addition, the study group was a heterogeneous group of patients with respect to corticosteroid indication.

The large patient cohort was powered sufficiently (significance level $P = .05$, 95% power) to

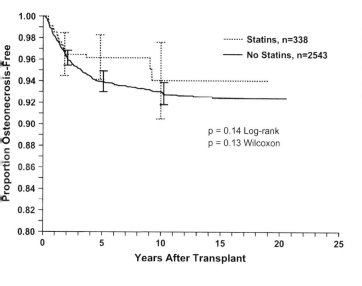

Fig. 1. A univariate Kaplan-Meier life table analysis of ON-free survival of kidney transplant patients on statins identified no trend in ON risk reduction for patients taking statins ($P = .14$, log-rank). Error bars = 95% confidence intervals.

Table 2
Cox multivariate analysis table of predictors with relative risk

Predictor	Adjusted Relative Risk (95% CI)	P Value
Gender (as male)	1.52 (1.11–2.09)	0.008
Number of rejection episodes	1.17 (1.04–1.32)	0.009
Year of transplant	0.96 (0.93–0.99)	0.01
Statin use	1.08 (0.61–1.91)	0.8

detect a reduction in risk as small as 3% at 5 years and 5% at 10 years in the incidences of ON. The authors did not identify any risk reduction; therefore, given the definition of statin exposure, if a reduction in ON incidence exists it is likely less than 5% at 10 years. The authors believe a reduction of risk of 5% or less is of dubious clinical importance.

The number of rejection episodes, a surrogate of peak-corticosteroid exposure, was associated with the development of ON. This would be expected, given the body of knowledge identifying a relationship between corticosteroids and ON. As all of the patients were on corticosteroid immunosuppression, the authors could not study if actual corticosteroid exposure was related to ON development. However, the data demonstrated that a higher number of rejection episodes was associated with a higher incidence of ON.

The data also suggest that male gender is associated with an increased risk (34%) of ON when compared with females. To the authors' knowledge, this has not been reported previously. The explanation for this finding is unknown, yet a gender difference related to differing fat metabolism may be a factor.[27,28]

The present study has some limitations. The methodology is suboptimal because it is not a randomized prospective study; however, the large size of the patient cohort and the statistical significance achieved support the validity of the results and conclusion. Some of the patients assigned to the nonstatin group actually had some limited exposure to statins, but not enough to meet the specific defined criteria for this study. The definition for statin usage was delineated to identify those patients who were taking statins at the time of highest risk for developing ON. Therefore, although the nonstatin group is not a pure nonstatin group, its composition is justified biologically. Asymptomatic patients with ON were not captured, as most of the cases were self-reported and prospective MRI screening was not done routinely. Although prevalence of asymptomatic ON has been reported between 6% and 9% in

various studies,[29–31] and the detection of asymptomatic disease is interesting, it is unlikely to change a patient's disease management. Fortunately, asymptomatic disease tends to have a benign course in the majority of patients.[29,30] In some rare cases, spontaneous resolution has been documented.[32]

This study included only renal transplant patients, so the data may or may not be applicable to patients at risk for ON for other reasons. While it would have been useful to analyze the relationship between cholesterol levels and ON, the authors did not have sufficient data on cholesterol levels to perform such an analysis; however, dosages were modified in principle to reduce cholesterol to clinically appropriate levels. All statins may not be the same. Nevertheless, the authors are not aware of data to suggest that therapeutic dosages of different statins have a variable influence on the pathophysiology of ON. Finally, as all of the patients were on corticosteroid immunosuppression, the authors could not study if actual corticosteroid exposure was related to ON development. The authors believe that the large size and homogeneity of the patient cohort, from a single transplant center, with the prospective collection of data, partially offset these deficiencies. Despite the stated limitations of this study, the data and analysis provides important new information in our knowledge of ON, and it is unlikely that a randomized, prospective study will be performed to address this study's goal.

The authors conclude that among renal transplant patients, statin usage does not appear to lower the risk of ON. Large-scale, randomized trials might reveal a reduced incidence of ON related to statin usage, but it is unlikely to be very large. The number of rejection episodes and male gender was associated with a higher risk.

ACKNOWLEDGMENTS

The authors thank Paul Lender for all the figures and data management.

REFERENCES

1. Harrington KD, Murray WR, Kountz SL, et al. Avascular necrosis of bone after renal transplantation. J Bone Joint Surg Am 1971;53(2):203–15.

2. Ibels LS, Alfrey AC, Huffer WE, et al. Aseptic necrosis of bone following renal transplantation: experience in 194 transplant recipients and review of the literature. Medicine (Baltimore) 1978;57(1):25–45.

3. Julian BA, Quarles LD, Niemann KM. Musculoskeletal complications after renal transplantation: pathogenesis and treatment. Am J Kidney Dis 1992;19(2): 99–120.

4. Carvalho AC, Lees RS, Vaillancourt RA, et al. Intravascular coagulation in hyperlipidemia. Thromb Res 1976;8(6):843–57.

5. Jones JP Jr. Fat embolism, intravascular coagulation, and osteonecrosis. Clin Orthop Relat Res 1993;(292):294–308.

6. Saito S, Ohzono K, Ono K. Early arteriopathy and postulated pathogenesis of osteonecrosis of the femoral head. The intracapital arterioles. Clin Orthop Relat Res 1992;(277):98–110.

7. Hedri H, Cherif M, Zouaghi K, et al. Avascular osteonecrosis after renal transplantation. Transplant Proc 2007;39(4):1036–8.

8. Le Parc JM, Andre T, Helenon O, et al. Osteonecrosis of the hip in renal transplant recipients. Changes in functional status and magnetic resonance imaging findings over three years in three hundred five patients. Rev Rhum Engl Ed 1996;63(6):413–20.

9. Marston SB, Gillingham K, Bailey RF, et al. Osteonecrosis of the femoral head after solid organ transplantation: a prospective study. J Bone Joint Surg Am 2002;84-A(12):2145–51.

10. Arlet J. Nontraumatic avascular necrosis of the femoral head. Past, present, and future. Clin Orthop Relat Res 1992;(277):12–21.

11. Cruess RL. Osteonecrosis of bone. Current concepts as to etiology and pathogenesis. Clin Orthop Relat Res 1986;(208):30–9.

12. Mont MA, Hungerford DS. Non-traumatic avascular necrosis of the femoral head. J Bone Joint Surg Am 1995;77(3):459–74.

13. Cui Q, Wang GJ, Balian G. Steroid-induced adipogenesis in a pluripotential cell line from bone marrow. J Bone Joint Surg Am 1997;79(7):1054–63.

14. Cui Q, Wang GJ, Su CC, et al. The Otto Aufranc Award. Lovastatin prevents steroid induced adipogenesis and osteonecrosis. Clin Orthop Relat Res 1997;(344):8–19.

15. Li X, Jin L, Cui Q, et al. Steroid effects on osteogenesis through mesenchymal cell gene expression. Osteoporos Int 2005;16(1):101–8.

16. Li X, Cui Q, Kao C, et al. Lovastatin inhibits adipogenic and stimulates osteogenic differentiation by suppressing PPARgamma2 and increasing Cbfa1/Runx2 expression in bone marrow mesenchymal cell cultures. Bone 2003;33(4):652–9.

17. Pritchett JW. Statin therapy decreases the risk of osteonecrosis in patients receiving steroids. Clin Orthop Relat Res 2001;(386):173–8.

18. Wang GJ, Cui Q, Balian G. The Nicolas Andry Award. The pathogenesis and prevention of steroid-induced osteonecrosis. Clin Orthop Relat Res 2000;(370):295–310.

19. Humar A, Johnson EM, Gillingham KJ, et al. Venous thromboembolic complications after kidney and kidney-pancreas transplantation: a multivariate analysis. Transplantation 1998;65(2):229–34.

20. Almond PS, Matas A, Gillingham K, et al. Risk factors for chronic rejection in renal allograft recipients. Transplantation 1993;55(4):752–6 [discussion: 756–7].

21. Cox D. The analysis of exponentially distributed lifetimes with two types of failures. J R Stat Soc 1959; 21(series B):411–21.

22. Kaplan EL, Meier P. Nonparametric estimation for incomplete observations. J Am Stat Assoc 1958; 53:457–81.

23. Maritz FJ, Conradie MM, Hulley PA, et al. Effect of statins on bone mineral density and bone histomorphometry in rodents. Arterioscler Thromb Vasc Biol 2001;21(10):1636–41.

24. Jacobs B. Epidemiology of traumatic and nontraumatic osteonecrosis. Clin Orthop Relat Res 1978;(130):51–67.

25. Ono K, Tohjima T, Komazawa T. Risk factors of avascular necrosis of the femoral head in patients with systemic lupus erythematosus under high-dose corticosteroid therapy. Clin Orthop Relat Res 1992;(277):89–97.

26. Zizic TM, Marcoux C, Hungerford DS, et al. Corticosteroid therapy associated with ischemic necrosis of bone in systemic lupus erythematosus. Am J Med 1985;79(5):596–604.

27. Lima JJ, Mauras N, Kissoon N, et al. Influence of sex and beta2 adrenergic receptor haplotype on resting and terbutaline-stimulated whole body lipolysis. Metabolism 2005;54(4):492–9.

28. Mittendorfer B. Sexual dimorphism in human lipid metabolism. J Nutr 2005;135(4):681–6.

29. Fordyce MJ, Solomon L. Early detection of avascular necrosis of the femoral head by MRI. J Bone Joint Surg Br 1993;75(3):365–7.

30. Mulliken BD, Renfrew DL, Brand RA, et al. Prevalence of previously undetected osteonecrosis of the femoral head in renal transplant recipients. Radiology 1994;192(3):831–4.

31. Tervonen O, Mueller DM, Matteson EL, et al. Clinically occult avascular necrosis of the hip: prevalence in an asymptomatic population at risk. Radiology 1992;182(3):845–7.

32. Cheng EY, Thongtrangan I, Laorr A, et al. Spontaneous resolution of osteonecrosis of the femoral head. J Bone Joint Surg Am 2004;86-A(12):2594–9.

Bone Marrow Edema Syndrome in Postpartal Women: Treatment with Iloprost

Nicholas Aigner, MD*, Roland Meizer, MD, Dominik Meraner, MD, Stephan Becker, MD, Elizabeth Meizer, MD, Franz Landsiedl, MD

KEYWORDS

- Bone marrow edema syndrome
- Pregnancy • Iloprost • Therapy

Bone marrow edema syndrome (BMES) of the femoral head is a rarely seen disease in pregnant women, characterized by disabling pain in the hip without prior trauma, by a typical signal pattern on MRI, and by striking radiographic evidence of osteopenia limited to the hip.

The exact pathogenesis of BMES remains unclear. Commonly discussed theories include abnormalities of vascular factors, altered lipid metabolism, and decreased fibrinolysis in pregnant women with increased plasminogen activator inhibitor-1 and lowered antithrombin-III activities.[1–3] Furthermore, thromboembolism (eg, caused by the Shwartzman reaction), obstruction of arteriolar inflow or venous outflow, or injury to the vessel wall caused by vasculitis, may lead to BMES[2–5] or osteonecrosis (ON).[5,6] Besides this, a hemolysis-elevated-liver-enzymes-and-low-platelet-count (HELLP) syndrome may occur in 25% of patients who develop gestosis, which is characterized by activation of the coagulation mechanisms and bone marrow alterations up to ON. The risk of ON is even more elevated when corticosteroids are associated for HELLP treatment.[7] In general, serum corticosteroid levels are elevated threefold in pregnant women as compared with nonpregnant women.[8] As in the nonpregnant population, most of pregnancy-associated BMES or ON in pregnant women is localized to the femoral head because of presumed anatomic and biomechanical reasons.

Different therapeutic attempts have been made to provide relief of pain or accelerate the natural course of healing in BMES.[5,9,10] The standard treatment of BMES consists of analgesic medications in combination with reduced weight-bearing and physical therapy. Better results regarding pain management are achieved by surgical intervention, with core decompression being the current gold standard.[5,11] In recent studies, parenteral administration of the vasoactive prostacyclin analog iloprost has been presented as an alternative therapy.[12–14]

The authors' objective was to assess the effect of a pharmacologic agent with broad activity spectrum ranging from local action of the terminal vascular bed to platelet aggregation.[15] This was done through a prospective pilot study in six pregnant women with BMES.

MATERIALS AND METHODS

Six subjects (eight hips) with MRI findings characteristic for BMES of the femoral head were included in this prospective pilot study. The subjects (age 30 to 43 years, mean age 38 years) presented with pain on effort with gait disturbance, and pain at rest starting in the last 3 months of pregnancy at a mean gestational age of 29 weeks (25 to 32 weeks). Symptoms rapidly progressed over a 2-week period in all cases. Two subjects

Orthopedic Hospital Vienna Speising, Speisingerstrasse 109, 1130 Vienna, Austria
* Corresponding author.
E-mail address: nicolas.aigner@oss.at (N. Aigner).

Orthop Clin N Am 40 (2009) 241–247
doi:10.1016/j.ocl.2008.10.007

with bilateral hip pain showed unilateral onset with symptoms with a contralateral progression after 3 weeks. Two subjects were initially misdiagnosed as pregnancy-associated lumbalgia. No trauma, alcohol abuse, or corticosteroid medication was reported. Five subjects were primiparous and one quintiparous. No family disposition was found in the subjects. MRI diagnoses were performed prepartum. All hips presented with BMES on MRI without a demarcated area or obvious damage to cartilage. Five subjects had normal deliveries and one had a caesarian section.

The subjects were treated with intravenous iloprost infusions in an off-label use. Iloprost (20 mcrg) (Bayer Schering Pharma AG, Germany) was given for 6 hours a day on 5 consecutive days, beginning 10 days after parturition.[5–14]

As breast-feeding is contraindicated for this treatment, the milk was discarded for a period of 1 week—that is, two days longer than the intravenous regimen—and the newborn infants were fed with substitutive milk for this time. This range of time was considered sufficient, as the half-life of elimination of iloprost is biphasic at 4 and 34 minutes. One subject did not restart breastfeeding after this period.

To evaluate MRI changes, coronal and sagittal T1-weighted spin echo sequences and short-tau inverted recovery (STIR) sequences were performed before and 12 weeks after the onset of therapy. Plain anteroposterior and lateral weight-bearing radiographs were performed postpartum. Pain at rest and effort-induced pain were assessed by the subjects at each visit during the study and follow-up using a 10-cm visual analog scale (VAS).

RESULTS
Baseline Characteristics of Participants

Treatment before this study consisted of oral paracetamol in three subjects for a mean period of 6 weeks (without notable effect on their symptoms), and reduction of weight-bearing (half-body weight up to nonweight bearing) in all patients for 3 to 10 weeks. Two subjects showed mild hypercholesterolemia and hypertriglyceridemia, two subjects a slightly elevated blood sedimentation rate, and one subject a mildly elevated C-reactive protein. No further abnormalities were seen in the various blood parameters. MRI revealed BMES of the whole femoral head and the neck of the affected hips, with absence of a demarcated necrotic bone area. Plain radiographs performed after birth in two subjects (three hips) displayed a slight regional osteopenia of the femoral head and neck; the other four cases (five hips) were normal. The pain level of all subjects did not change in the affected hips after birth but before treatment.

Clinical and MRI Course

All six subjects improved immediately during the first 2 weeks after the beginning of the intravenous therapy. The severity of pain at rest (VAS) decreased from a mean of 44 mm (range, 23 mm–56 mm) to 2 mm (range, 0 mm–4 mm) after 1 month and to 1 mm (range, 0 mm–3 mm) after 3 months. The severity of pain on effort was reduced from a mean of 54 mm (range, 33 mm–74 mm) to 6 mm (range, 0 mm–12 mm) after 1 month and to 3 mm (range, 0 mm–8 mm) after 3 months (**Fig. 1**). All patients presented complete functional recovery of the hips starting in the first through the last follow-up (14–43, average 31 months) after therapy. No new episodes of BMES occurred.

MRI follow-up after 3 months showed that the BMES had disappeared in five subjects (7 hips) and subtotal regression with a small area of residual edema was found in the femoral neck in one pain-free subject with bilateral affection (**Figs. 2 and 3**). No progression to ON was seen in the cohort at last follow-up.

Side Effects

Adverse events during treatment were seen in four subjects who complained of mild headache and flush during the first infusion, which disappeared immediately after the end of each infusion. No serious adverse events were observed and no subject had to discontinue the treatment prematurely.

DISCUSSION

BMES was first described in 1959, by Curtiss and Kincaid,[16] as a clinical syndrome characterized by

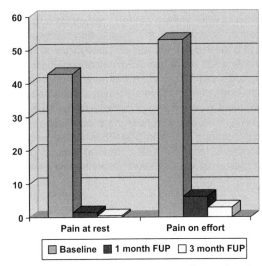

Fig. 1. Course of pain at rest and on effort at baseline and 1- and 3-months follow-up after iloprost therapy

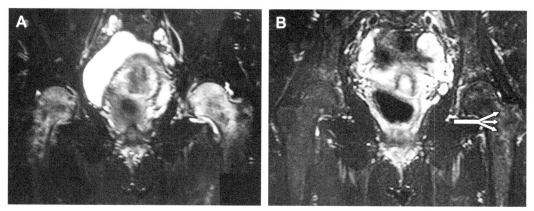

Fig. 2. (*A*) T2-weighted fat-suppressed MRI with bilateral BMES of the femoral head and neck before therapy in a 38-year-old subject. The head of the fetus is visible. (*B*) Ten weeks after therapy: complete restitution of the right side and a minimal residual BMES of the femoral neck of the left side (*arrows*).

hip pain, reduced bone density in plain radiographs, and spontaneous regression of symptoms in women during the last trimester of pregnancy. The majority of BMES occurs around the hip and, less frequently, at the knee. Pain is caused by an increased intraosseous pressure (normal 20 mm Hg–30 mm Hg). Effusion and a limited range of motion are not always present and not specific.[6] Standard laboratory values are usually normal or nonspecific. Patients usually do not show the typical risk factors for osteonecrosis, such as massive alcohol consumption or

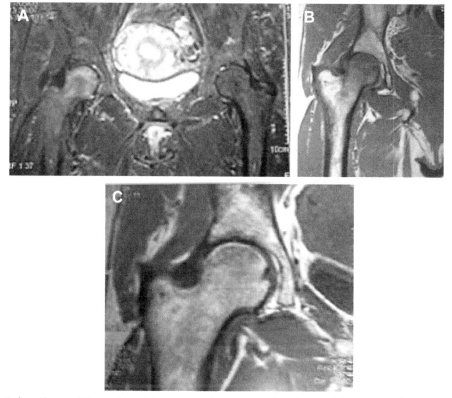

Fig. 3. (*A*) Before-therapy T2-weighted fat suppressed sequences of a 41-year-old woman with BMES of the right femoral head and the superior part of the femoral head. The left hip shows a normal signal pattern. The fetus is visible. (*B*) T1-weighted MRI of the right hip before therapy. (*C*) T1-weighted MRI of the right hip 3 months after therapy with iloprost, showing complete remission of the BMES.

corticosteroid therapy. Plain radiographs occasionally reveal local osteopenia in the area affected by BMES, but structural changes of this type are manifested late. The final diagnosis of BMES is established by MRI, which shows a typical signal pattern. BMES shows high signal intensity on T1-weighted images and a low signal intensity on T2-weighted images, especially when fat-suppressed sequences are applied (STIR).[17] Enhancement of BMES lesions after parenteral administration of contrast agents indicates hypervascularity and repair activity. The abnormal signal in MRI is not caused by fluid alone. Histologic analyses have shown a varying amount of intra- and extracellular fluid accumulation in the bone-marrow cavities, fat cell destruction as an expression of marrow necrosis, as well as formation of new bone and fibrovascular regeneration.[5,18] The number of trabeculae is normal but bone-mineral density is decreased.[19]

Several investigators have reported a relationship between transient BMES and ON,[6,20,21] but the incidence of progression from BMES to ON is still unclear. The typical characteristics of BMES and ON are summarized in **Table 1**. Furthermore, there is still controversy as to whether ischemic BMES represents a distinct self-limiting disease[1,22,23] or a type of reflex-sympathetic dystrophy.[9,24]

Various treatment options of BMES have been reported. These include surgical treatments, such as core decompression.[5,11,25–27] This surgical method has been recommended for rapid and complete reduction of symptoms, with a return to normal MR signal patterns, based on the theory that pain in the BMES and ON is caused by elevated intramedullary pressure.

Radke and colleagues[25] investigated a collective of 43 subjects with BMES of the hip, in which five were treated with nonsteroidal anti-inflammatory drugs and limited weight-bearing, and 38 were treated by core decompression followed by limited weight-bearing. Both groups had the same clinical outcome. Core decompression enabled a faster recovery than in the conservatively treated patients. There were no complications, but progression to osteonecrosis was seen in both groups.

In another study, the same group investigated 22 hips with BMES treated with core decompression. After an average of 7 days, all subjects were pain-free after the procedure. In two subjects, BMES progressed to ON despite core decompression. All others had no signal alterations of the head of the femur on MRI after 6 months. The postoperative Harris Hip Score in subjects with BMES had an average of 94 points.[26]

In a prospective study, Hofmann and colleagues[27] found an immediate relief of pain in 43 hip joints after surgery. The average duration of symptoms with conservative treatment could be dramatically reduced by core decompression from 5 months to 2 months.

Although core decompression has a low complication rate and can be performed as an outpatient procedure, proximal femoral fractures have been reported.[7,11] This complication can be avoided by the use of thin 2.2-mm or 2.5-mm k-wires instead of the traditional 8-mm to 10-mm hollow trephines.[28] Up to 6 weeks of partial or complete weight-bearing are recommended after core decompression. Symptomatic nonsurgical treatments (reduction of weight bearing, analgesic and anti-inflammatory medication, physiotherapy) may take as much as 6 to 12 months for full recovery.

With regard to pharmacologic treatment of BMES, the bisphosphonate alendronate (orally applied in the dosage of 70 mg per week in combination with vitamin D and calcium supplement) as well as risedronate were investigated in several studies in the last few years.[29,30] The supposed mechanism of action of these agents in the therapy of BMES is an inhibition of bone resorption, an increased bone remodeling, and a raised bone-mineral density. In a study of 12 subjects with BMES, ibandronate was administered as an initial 4-mg intravenous dose with a second, optional injection of 2 mg at 3 months. Daily calcium and vitamin D supplements were provided. Intravenous ibandronate provided rapid and substantial pain relief. The mean VAS score decreased from 8.4 at baseline to 0.5 at 6 months, at which time seven subjects had achieved complete pain relief.[29] Alendronate was able to decrease the pain and the BME and increased the functional outcome in postmenopausal women with gonarthrosis.[30]

The off-label application of the vasoactive prostacyclin analog iloprost for the treatment of painful BMES has been investigated in previous studies.[12–14,31] This substance is registered for therapy of critical ischemia secondary to peripheral atherosclerotic disease or diabetic angiopathy. The substance dilates arterioles and venoles, reduces capillary permeability, and inhibits thrombocyte aggregation. Apart from this local impact on rheologic properties of the terminal vascular bed, it diminishes the concentration of oxygen radicals and leukotrienes. In clincal use, the most frequent side effects of this substance are headache, nausea, and flush. Administration is contraindicated in pregnant patients, in patients anticoagulated with warfarin or heparin, in cases of concomitant gastrointestinal ulcers, and in patients with heart insufficiency, recent myocardial infarction, or unstable

Table 1
Characteristics of bone marrow edema syndrome and osteonecrosis

	BMES	ON
Pathophysiology	Diffuse reversible ischemia of epi- and metaphyseal bone	Localized subchondral ischemia of epiphysis by occlusion of the arterial inflow, venous outflow, intravascular occlusion (fat embolia, sickle cell anemia), extravascular tamponade of the sinusoids
Bilateral affection	Up to 50%	40%–70%
Risk factors	In most patients, none; pregnancy	Pregnancy, alcohol, corticosteroids, sickle cell anemia, Gaucher, Caisson's disease, hyperlipidemia
Natural course	Self-limiting after 6 to 12 months, progression to ON discussed,	Progressing in stages ending with collapse of the affected bone and destruction of the joint
Histology	Intra- and extracellular fluid accumulation in bone marrow cavities, fat-cell destruction, fibrovascular regeneration, decreased bone mineral density, no diminution of trabeculae	Necrosis of osteoblasts, osteoclasts, and osteocytes, empty lacunae, resorption of necrotic trabeculae, sclerosis of margin of necrotic to vital bone, bone marrow edema, fat cell destruction, fibrovascular regeneration
Radiography	Initially normal signal, diffuse demineralization after weeks ("transient osteoporosis")	Early normal signal pattern, later demarcation of necrotic bone, curvi-linear lucent line parallel to the cortical margin because of insufficiency fractures ("crescent sign"), impaction of subchondral bone, later collapse of the bone and secondary osteoarthritis
MRI	Early detection possible, low signal intensity on T1-weighted images, high signal intensity on T2-weighted fat-suppressed images	Demarcated area of necrotic bone ("double line sign"), MRI crescent sign, signs of BMES, later impaction of the subchondral bone with flattening of the femoral head, narrowing of the joint gap, affection of the acetabulum
Clinical course	Abrupt or gradual onset of pain, pain during activity and frequently at rest and at night, slightly restricted range of motion	Abrupt or gradual onset of pain during activity and frequently at rest and at night, in later stages massive restriction of range of motion and mobility

angina pectoris. Rapid pain reduction and accelerated normalization of MR patterns were reported in several studies in different joints of adults, children, and adolescents.[12–14,31] The rationale of therapy with iloprost was of a pharmacologic agent acting as vasodilator on all parts of the terminal vascular bed.

In a previous study, subjects with BMES in the femoral head after core decompression were compared with parenteral application of iloprost over 5 consecutive days.[14] Both groups showed a rapid remission of the clinical symptoms. All subjects in the iloprost group demonstrated complete restitution of MRI patterns after 3 months. The surgical group still showed a residual edema in 4 out of 20 hips in the same time period.

In a double-blind, randomized study investigating 41 subjects with painful bone marrow edema of the knee, oral application of iloprost (up to 300 mcrg per day) was tested versus tramadol (up to 300 mg per day). The treatment duration was 4 weeks. The Larson knee score was used to assess function before and during treatment and 3 months after the start of treatment. MRI of the affected knees were obtained before and 3 months afterwards. In both groups, no significant differences were found regarding analgesic effect and improvement of functional assessment. A statistically significant regression of BME was only seen in the study group treated with iloprost.[31]

There are only a few publications about BMES of pregnant women, which are mostly case reports and small series.[19,32,33] Those subjects were treated conservatively with restricted weight-bearing, analgesic drugs, and physiotherapy, and showed remission of symptoms at 4 to 10 months, which does not differ from nonpregnant patients with BMES of the femoral head. In a study[17] of 7 subjects, rapid decrease of BMES following core decompression was demonstrated. In two subjects, treated conservatively, markedly delayed healing was evident. In the current study, most subjects showed rapid improvement of symptoms and normalization of hip function, which was maintained throughout the observation period. This indicates that there is analgesic capacity of iloprost in the treatment of BMES.

As proposed by Boos and colleagues,[9] MRI was performed 12 weeks after treatment. Because of the general contraindication of iloprost in pregnant and breastfeeding women, the authors recommend starting the off-label use of iloprost only about 1 week after delivery and to discard the milk for 7 days after the first infusion. This regimen is continued two days longer than the infusion therapy so that the drug is completely eliminated from the maternal circulation, and the subjects can safely start breastfeeding again.

Limitations of this study are certainly the small number of subjects, the absence of a control group, and the short follow-up period. Nevertheless, it is important to be aware of this condition as part of the differential diagnosis of hip, groin, or low back pain in pregnant women in the last 3 months of pregnancy to avoid aggressive and unnecessary diagnostic and therapeutic procedures. Therefore, an early MRI diagnostic is recommended that can easily and safely be performed during pregnancy.

SUMMARY

The parenteral administration of the vasoactive drug iloprost represents a new approach for the treatment of painful BMES of the hip in pregnant women. Relief from pain, restoration of functional capacity, and normalization of the MRI signal pattern can be achieved quickly, thus avoiding the need for surgical intervention. As the substance is contraindicated during pregnancy, therapy may begin after parturition with a short discontinuation of breastfeeding. Further double-blind, randomized, and controlled investigations are required to substantiate these findings.

REFERENCES

1. Berger CE, Kroner AH, Minai-Pour MB, et al. Biochemical markers of bone metabolism in bone marrow edema syndrome of the hip. Bone 2003; 33:346–51.
2. Glueck CJ, Freiberg R, Glueck HI, et al. Hypofibrinolysis: a common, major cause of osteonecrosis. Am J Hematol 1994;45:156–66.
3. Glueck CJ, Freiberg R, Glueck HI, et al. Idiopathic osteonecrosis, hypofibrinolysis, high plasminogen activator inhibitor, high lipoprotein(a), and therapy with stanozolol. Am J Hematol 1995;48(4):213–20.
4. Atsumi T, Kuroki Y. Role of impairment of blood supply of the femoral head in the pathogenesis of idiopathic osteonecrosis. Clin Orthop 1992;277: 22–30.
5. Veldhuizen PJ, Neff J, Murphey MD, et al. Decreased fibrinolytic potential in patients with idiopathic avascular necrosis and transient osteoporosis of the hip. Am J Hematol 1993;44:243–8.
6. Hofmann S, Engel A, Neuhold A, et al. Bone marrow oedema syndrome and transient osteoporosis of the hip. J Bone Joint Surg Br 1993;75-B:210–6.
7. Jager M, Wild A, Krauspe R, et al. Osteonecrosis and HELLP-syndrome. Z Geburtshilfe Neonatol 2003;207:213–9.
8. Genez BM, Wilson MR, Houk RW, et al. Early osteonecrosis of the femoral head: detection in high-risk patients with MR-imaging. Radiology 1988;168: 521–4.
9. Boos S, Sigmund G, Huhle P, et al. MR of transient osteoporosis. Primary diagnosis and follow-up after treatment. Fortschr Roentgenstr 1993;158:201–6.
10. Lakhanpal S, Ginsburg WW, Luthra HS, et al. Transient regional osteoporosis. A study of 56 cases and review of the literature. Ann Intern Med 1987; 106:444–50.
11. Aigner N, Eberl V, Schneider W, et al. Effect of core decompression in early stages of necrosis of the femoral head—an MRI-controlled study. Int Orthop 2002;26:31–5.
12. Meizer R, Radda C, Stolz G, et al. MRI-controlled retrospective analysis of 104 patients with bone marrow edema of different localisations treated with lloprost. Wien Klin Wochenschr 2005;117: 278–86.
13. Petje G, Radler C, Aigner N, et al. Aseptic osteonecrosis in childhood: diagnosis and treatment. Orthopade 2002;31:1027–36.

14. Aigner N, Petje G, Schneider W, et al. Bone marrow oedema syndrome of the femoral head: comparison of therapy with the prostacycline-analogue iloprost and core decompression. Wien Klin Wochenschr 2005;117:130–5.

15. Grant SM, Goa KL. Iloprost—a review of its pharmacodynamic and pharmacokinetic properties, and therapeutic potential in peripheral vascular disease, myocardial ischaemia and extracorporal circulation procedures. Drugs 1992;43:889–924.

16. Curtiss PH Jr, Kincaid WE. Transitory demineralization of the hip in pregnancy: a report of three cases. J Bone Joint Surg Am 1959;41-A:1327–33.

17. Kramer J, Hofmann S, Engel A, et al. Necrosis of the head of femur and bone marrow edema syndrome in pregnancy. Fortschr Roentgenstr 1993;159:126–31.

18. Plenk H Jr, Hofmann S, Eschberger J, et al. Histomorphology and bone morphometry of the bone marrow edema of the hip. Clin Orthop 1997;334:73–84.

19. Funk JL, Shoback DM, Genant HK, et al. Transient osteoporosis of the hip in pregnancy: natural history of changes in bone mineral density. Clin Endocrinol 1995;43:373–82.

20. Hauzeur JP, Perlmutter N, Appelboom T, et al. Medullary impairment at an early stage of non-traumatic osteonecrosis of the femoral head. Rheumatol Int 1991;11:215–7.

21. Staudenherz A, Hofmann S, Breitenseher M, et al. Diagnostic patterns for bone marrow oedema syndrome and avascular necrosis of the femoral head in dynamic bone scintigraphy. Nucl Med Commun 1997;18:1178–88.

22. Froberg PK, Braunstein EM, Buckwalter KA, et al. Osteonecrosis, transient osteoporosis, and transient bone marrow edema. Radiol Clin North Am 1996;34:273–91.

23. Krause R, Glas K, Schulz A, et al. The transitory bone marrow edema syndrome of the hip. Z Orthop Ihre Grenzgeb 2002;140:286–96.

24. Doury P. Bone marrow oedema, transient osteoporosis and algodystrophy. J Bone Joint Surg Br 1994; 76-B:993–4.

25. Radke S, Kirschner S, Seipel V, et al. Treatment of transient bone marrow oedema of the hip—a comparative study. Int Orthop 2003;27(3):149–52.

26. Radke S, Rader C, Kenn W, et al. Transient marrow edema syndrome of the hip: results after core decompression. A prospective MRI-controlled study in 22 patients. Arch Orthop Trauma Surg 2003; 123(5):223–7.

27. Hofmann S, Schneider W, Breitenseher M, et al. "Transient osteoporosis" as a special reversible form of femur head necrosis. Orthopade 2000; 29(5):411–9.

28. Rader CP. Transient osteoporosis and osteonecrosis of the femoral head. Risk factors, classification and differential diagnosis. Orthopade 2007;36(5):423–9.

29. Ringe JD, Dorst A, Faber H, et al. Effective and rapid treatment of painful localized transient osteoporosis (bone marrow edema) with intravenous ibandronate. Osteoporos Int 2005;16(12):2063–8.

30. Carbone LD, Nevitt MC, Wildy K, et al. The relationship of antiresorbtive drug use to structural findings and symptoms of knee osteoarthritis. Arthritis Rheum 2004;52(5):1622–3.

31. Mayerhoefer ME, Kramer J, Breitenseher MJ, et al. Short-term outcome of painful bone marrow oedema of the knee following oral treatment with iloprost or tramadol: results of an exploratory phase II study of 41 patients. Rheumatology (Oxford) 2007;46(9): 1460–5 [Epub 2007 Jul 17].

32. Sweeney AT, Blake M, Holick MF, et al. Transient osteoporosis of the hip in pregnancy. J Clin Densitom 2000;3:291–7.

33. Uematsu N, Nakayama Y, Shirai Y, et al. Transient osteoporosis of the hip during pregnancy. J Nippon Med Sch 2000;67:459–63.

Assessment of Bone Perfusion with Contrast-Enhanced Magnetic Resonance Imaging

Jonathan H. Lee, MD[a], Jonathan P. Dyke, PhD[b],
Douglas Ballon, PhD[b], Deborah McK. Ciombor, PhD[c],
Glenn Tung, MD[d], Roy K. Aaron, MD[c],*

KEYWORDS

- Osteoarthritis • MRI • Animal model
- Guinea pig • Subchondral • Venous outflow occlusion

The pathophysiology of osteoarthritis (OA) and avascular necrosis (AVN) remains unknown. In both cases, the late pathology of the disease is clear, but the events that lead up to ultimate joint degeneration are not well understood. Usually the disease is not discovered until late in its course, when only surgical or palliative methods are available. Early detection could allow for targeting of aspects of the disease pathophysiology and thus alter or stop the course of the disease. Recent work suggested that OA and AVN may have early vascular components that change underlying bone perfusion in the affected bone and joint and contribute to the clinical cascade of each disease.[1,2] Measuring blood flow in bone in the region of a synovial joint is difficult, particularly if it is to be done in a noninvasive manner. Invasive techniques exist, such as radioactive microsphere methods, but availability of technology for such techniques precludes their use in humans.[3] We have applied a technique to assess bone perfusion

by noninvasive methods to study the vascular components of OA and AVN.

Dynamic contrast-enhanced MRI (DCE-MRI), a technique initially used in brain imaging, can be used as a way to quantify bone perfusion accurately and noninvasively in a synovial joint. This method uses a standard MRI contrast agent (Gd-DTPA) and is easily and safely performed in laboratory animals and humans. Changes in bone perfusion are related to bone marrow edema, a common clinical finding seen in MRI. The presence of bone marrow edema is widespread and is seen in many entities, such as trauma, OA, and AVN. Numerous clinical studies have associated bone marrow edema—or bone marrow lesions as they are sometimes called—with pain, bone remodeling, and cartilage degeneration.[4] The causes of the marrow signal changes of edema seen on MRI and the pathologic significance of the MRI finding of bone marrow edema are uncertain.[5] It is thought that bone marrow

a Department of Orthopaedic Surgery, Columbia University Medical Center, 622 West 168th Street, PH 1130, New York, NY 10032, USA
b Citigroup Biomedical Imaging Center, Weill Medical College of Cornell University, 1300 York Avenue - Box 234, New York, NY 10021, USA
c Department of Orthopaedics, The Warren Alpert Medical School of Brown University, 100 Butler Drive, Providence, RI 02906, USA
d Department of Radiology, The Warren Alpert Medical School of Brown University, Rhode Island Hospital, 593 Eddy Street, Providence, RI 02903, USA
* Corresponding author. Department of Orthopaedics, The Warren Alpert Medical School of Brown University, 100 Butler Drive, Providence, RI 02906, USA.
E-mail address: roy_aaron@brown.edu (R.K. Aaron).

Orthop Clin N Am 40 (2009) 249–257
doi:10.1016/j.ocl.2008.12.003
0030-5898/08/$ – see front matter © 2009 Elsevier Inc. All rights reserved.

orthopedic.theclinics.com

edema can be a marker of altered fluid dynamics and could indicate changes in intraosseous pressure and blood flow. Such changes in fluid dynamics are thought to drive the secretion of cytokines that contribute to the regulation of bone remodeling and cartilage degeneration. Traditional MRI is not capable of extracting such kinetic parameters as bone perfusion, but DCE-MRI is capable of extracting such data in a noninvasive way.

High signal intensity, as seen on T2-weighted images, signifies high water content; it is thought that bone marrow edema is a radiographic marker of increased intraosseous pressure and changes in blood flow. Intraosseous hypertension has been related to bone pain in several joints, and elevated intraosseous pressure has been observed in OA of the hip and knee.[6–8] Conventional contrast studies have demonstrated venous engorgement and stasis associated with intraosseous hypertension in OA of the hip.[8] Similar elevations of intraosseous pressure were found in patients with OA of the knee.[7] Patients without OA but with knee pain also exhibited intraosseous hypertension, but patients without OA and without pain had normal intraosseous pressures. Reduction of pressure by fenestration, or core decompression, is accompanied by a reduction in pain. Osteotomy of the proximal femur reduces intraosseous pressure and pain in patients with OA of the hip.[8] These observations collectively suggest that changes in fluid dynamics resulting in intraosseous hypertension are associated with bone pain and arthritis. These findings, coupled with bone marrow edema as seen on traditional MRI, lead us to use DCE-MRI to assess bone perfusion noninvasively.

This article describes a method for assessing bone perfusion with DCE-MRI in human patients and animals. By comparing the imaging data with histologic data, we demonstrate that regions of edema and decreased perfusion temporally precede and spatially co-localize with eventual cartilage degeneration, the final common pathway in OA and AVN.

METHODS

The use of DCE-MRI was evaluated in human patients and with an animal model. In human and animal studies, DCE-MRI was used; techniques were similar for the two groups. Specific techniques are described in detail elsewhere and are beyond the scope of this article.[9] In both cases, MRI data were acquired and dynamic perfusion data were extracted using mathematical modeling based on the Brix two-compartment pharmacokinetic

model.[10–12] In brief, the Brix two-compartment model is capable of producing perfusion parameters such as perfusion in to and out of a region of interest (eg, the region of subchondral bone adjacent to an arthritic joint). The rate of perfusion into such regions is also calculated.

Human data were collected from adult patients with painful bone marrow edema associated with OA or AVN. Each patient underwent a DCE-MRI scan for conditions such as infection, synovitis, fractures, and other conditions associated with bone marrow edema. Thirteen patients carried a diagnosis of OA, whereas 9 had AVN. The mean patient age was 52 (range, 22–92). Briefly, DCE-MRI was performed with a 1.5-T magnet using standard clinical coils. Gd-DTPA was injected by power-injector via large-bore peripheral intravenous line at a standard concentration of 0.1 mmol/kg. The focus of bone marrow edema was studied with eight continuous slices, 5 mm each. During data acquisition, TR was 5.5 and TE was 2.89. Data were obtained for 15 seconds after the injection initiation and collected every 10 seconds for the ensuing 5 minutes. Neighboring areas of nonedematous bone were used as internal controls.

Human data invariably are fraught with confounding factors, and longitudinal studies are difficult in humans. The Dunkin-Hartley guinea pig model is ideally suited to study the progression of OA. Histologically and biochemically, considerable resemblance exists between human and Dunkin-Hartley guinea pig OA. Just as in human OA, lesions appear preferentially on the medial aspect of the knee joint. The arthritis also develops spontaneously without any required surgical intervention, and the progression of arthritis over time has been well characterized.[13–15]

DCE-MRI was performed as reported elsewhere.[9] In brief, four different ages were selected (6 animals per group for a total of 24 animals) to study perfusion parameters at different stages of OA (6, 9, 12, and 15 months); these ages were selected based on well-characterized documentation of OA development.[13,16] All animals were acquired from Charles River Laboratories; central venous (jugular) catheters were surgically placed by staff there to ensure reliable venous access for Gd-DTPA perfusion studies. Imaging studies were conducted on a 3.0-T MRI. Data were acquired via a fast multiplanar spoiled gradient echo sequence with four to seven slices and a 12.1/3.8 ms TR/TE. A fast spin-echo short tau inversion recovery was also acquired to visualize bone marrow edema (TR = 6650 ms; TI = 180 ms; TE = 45 ms). The central line remained patent in all cases and was used to manually inject the

Gd-DTPA in all cases (0.3 mmol/kg). After all imaging was completed, animals were euthanized and tibias were harvested for measurement of subchondral bone thickness and histochemistry. Specimens were decalcified and prepared using Safranin-O/Fast Green stain. Histologic cartilage grade was assessed by the well-established method of Mankin.[17] Subchondral plate thickness was digitally measured at the central third of the medial and the lateral tibial plateaus. All data were analyzed as mean ± standard error of the mean (SEM); significance was determined by means of parametric and nonparametric tests, as was deemed appropriate based on the sample sizes and distributions.

RESULTS
Human Data

Sample regions of interest with associated time intensity curves are presented in **Fig. 1** (hip) and **Fig. 2** (knee). In both of these examples, note the difference in the shape of the curve on the right side of the figure (indicated by the red bar above the data curve in **Fig. 1**). Regions of edema are depicted with a continued rise in value over time, whereas regions without edema show decreased values over time. The later time points on these graphs are basically the "wash-out" phase for the contrast material. Failure to "wash out" can be interpreted as stasis or outflow obstruction. Such outflow obstruction was noted to be more extreme in the knee compared with the hip, possibly because of more contrasting anatomic regions (medial versus lateral femoral condyle or tibial plateau). Differences in morphology, infrastructure, and patterns of vascularization also can account for observed differences between the hip and the knee.

Data were pooled for the entire population, and pharmacokinetic modeling was used to extract quantitative parameters (**Table 1**). The three parameters are slope, amplitude (A), and perfusion out of the region of interest (k_{el}). Slope and amplitude were significantly greater in bone marrow edema compared with normal bone. Perfusion out of the region of interest was significantly lower in bone marrow edema compared with normal bone. The fact that k_{el} is lower in regions of bone marrow edema means that the edematous bone retains the Gd-DTPA to a greater degree and for a longer time than regions without edema, within the 5-minute scan time used in the experiments (**Fig. 3**).

If patients who have AVN are compared with patients who have OA, another phenomenon is found. As seen in **Fig. 4**, based on data from 13 patients who have OA and 9 patients who have AVN, decreased perfusion out of the region of interest is seen in AVN and OA, and the initial slope is the same. The amplitude is much lower in patients who have AVN compared with patients who have OA. This finding suggests that one might be able to differentiate between OA and AVN by using the amplitude of the time intensity curves. Why this difference was observed is unclear; it may be related to changes in capillary permeability in the regions of pathology.

Guinea Pig Data

Histologic changes observed in this study were consistent with previous reports described in the literature. **Fig. 5** presents histologic data and data reporting the subchondral bone thickness. Significant changes in histology were seen between the 9-month and 12-month time point, concomitant with an increase in subchondral plate thickness, also starting between the 9-month and 12-month time point. Sample time intensity curves are presented in **Fig. 6**. At 6 months of age, before significant OA was present, contrast dye did not collect and was seen to wash out over the course of the scan (as evidenced by the negative slope toward the end of the time intensity curves). At 12 months, OA occurred. This example was taken from a region of the medial tibial plateau in a region of subchondral bone below histologically significant OA. As evidenced by the persistent positive slope, the MRI contrast dye pooled in the region of interest, a finding that could be consistent with venous outflow obstruction.

Perfusion into the tibial plateau on the medial and the lateral sides remained constant at all time points. **Fig. 7** depicts outflow plotted with bone marrow edema. When these parameters are plotted together, one can see that changes in perfusion between the 6-month and the 9-month time points spatially co-localize and temporally precede changes in cartilage histology and bone remodeling in the medial tibial plateau.[18] These data are suggestive of a temporal and spatial relationship of edema to the eventual medial-sided cartilage and bone lesions of OA. Edema of the medial:lateral tibial plateau increased between 6 and 9 months of age but did not reach statistical significance ($P = .06$). Post-hoc power analysis demonstrated that with the same effect sizes and variances, statistical significance would be reached with a sample size of 12.

DISCUSSION

OA and AVN are common problems, both of which lead to joint degeneration, pain, and disability.

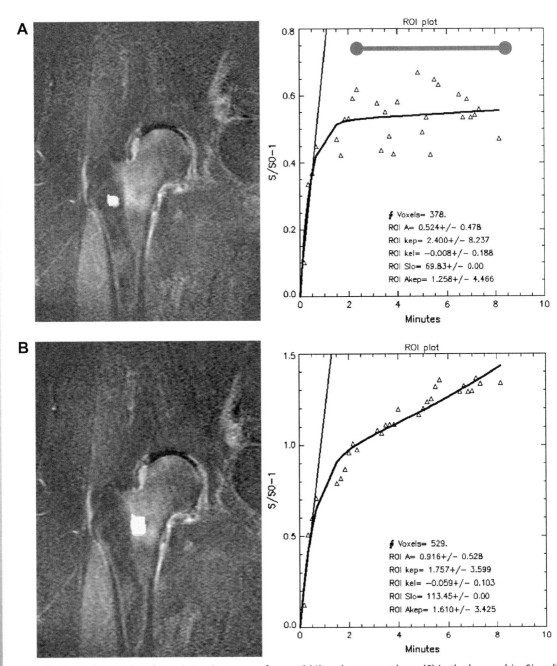

Fig. 1. Regions of interest and time intensity curves of normal (*A*) and marrow edema (*B*) in the human hip. Signal enhancement is observed in the proximal femur with bone marrow edema. Differences in amplitude, slope, and outflow are noted. The images are subtraction images showing enhancement at the end of the time course minus the baseline image intensity. The red bar above the data curve indicates the "wash-out" phase. (*From* Aaron RK, Dyke JP, Ciombor DM, et al. Perfusion abnormalities in subchondral bone associated with marrow edema, osteoarthritis, and avascular necrosis. Ann N Y Acad Sci 2007;1117:124–37; with permission.)

Early signs of both clinical entities may manifest as local changes in the fluid dynamics of the subchondral bone. Although this finding traditionally has been difficult to assess, we present a noninvasive method of using DCE-MRI to quantify changes in fluid dynamics. Human data and guinea pig data produced similar results. Regions of bone marrow edema demonstrated changes in perfusion, which may suggest venous outflow obstruction in the subchondral bone in areas of bone and cartilage pathology. Tsukamoto and colleagues[19] used similar DCE-MRI techniques in

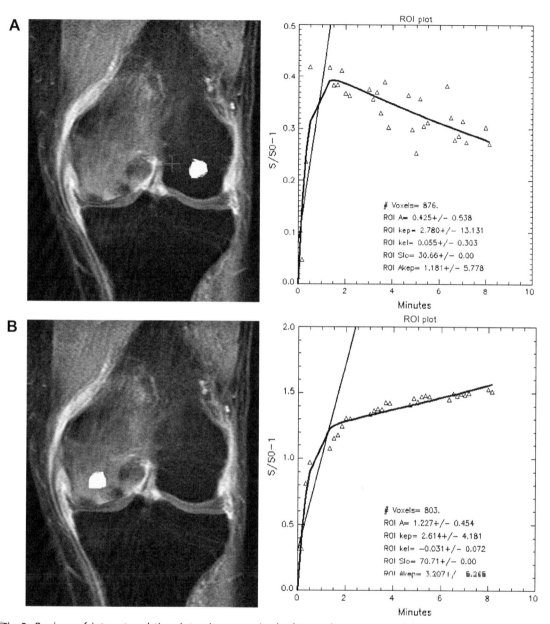

Fig. 2. Regions of interest and time intensity curves in the human knee in normal (*A*) and marrow edema (*B*) demonstrating signal enhancement with Gd-DTPA in the abnormal femoral condyle. Differences in amplitude, slope, and outflow are observed. (*From* Aaron RK, Dyke JP, Ciombor DM, et al. Perfusion abnormalities in subchondral bone associated with marrow edema, osteoarthritis, and avascular necrosis. Ann N Y Acad Sci 2007;1117:124–37; with permission.)

a canine model and validated their findings by using radioactive microsphere methods.

Our work with an animal model demonstrated that bone marrow edema lesions temporally precede changes in cartilage morphology and spatially localize at the site of eventual bone and cartilage lesions. Perfusion parameters extracted from our pharmacokinetic model point to outflow

obstruction as the primary change in kinetic parameters. Such outflow obstruction suggests increases in intraosseous pressure, which compound the problem of decreased perfusion. Estimated intraosseous pressure values can be extracted from our pharmacokinetic data; in humans, normal intraosseous pressure is 26 ± 3 mm Hg, whereas intraosseous pressure in OA is

Table 1
Data extracted using the pharmacokinetic model (mean ± SEM)

	Normal	Bone Marrow Edema	P Value
Slope	50 ± 7.1	95.2 ± 9.3	0.001
A	0.44 ± 0.06	0.99 ± 0.08	0.0001
k_{el}	0.09 ± 0.04	−0.04 ± 0.01	0.001

When compared with normal bone, slope was greater in subjects with bone marrow edema. Amplitude of the data (A) was also significantly greater by a factor of 2.5 in bone with marrow edema as compared with normal bone. The parameter indicating perfusion out of the region of interest, k_{el}, showed a negative value in patients with bone marrow edema as compared with a statistically significant positive value in normal bone.

43 ± 4 mm Hg.[20,21] Estimated value, in our human studies in regions of OA, is 45 mm Hg. Increased intraosseous pressure is one of the possible causative factors responsible for pain. This finding is of particular clinical interest because bone marrow edema or bone marrow lesions are commonly reported in numerous and varied clinical entities. They may exhibit the classic edema pattern observed after an anterior cruciate ligament tear or the chronic changes observed in end-stage OA. Such pharmacokinetic analysis may prove to be particularly useful if it is able to detect differences in perfusion characteristics in these different clinical scenarios.

The potential pathophysiologic significance of bone marrow edema is in its association with altered fluid dynamics in subchondral bone. Osteocytes secrete cytokines that regulate cartilage degeneration and bone remodeling, and osteocytes have been shown to change their cytokine expression profiles in response to changes in fluid flow, intraosseous pressure, and local oxygen availability. As determined in seminal studies performed by Arnoldi, increases in intraosseous

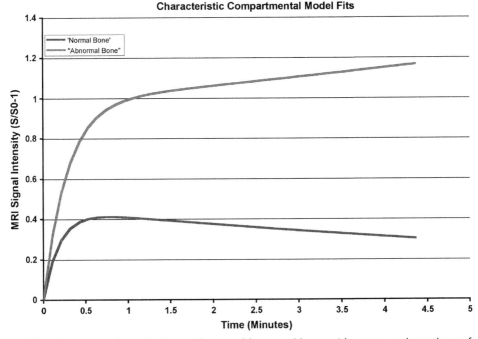

Fig. 3. Time intensity curves of populations with normal bone and bone with marrow edema drawn from the kinetic parameters in slope, A, and k_{el} representing inflow and outflow characteristics. Resolution of signal enhancement is beginning in normal bone by 3 to 4 minutes of scan time, whereas signal enhancement continues to rise in bone with marrow edema. This is interpreted as reflecting outflow obstruction and decreased perfusion (*From* Aaron RK, Dyke JP, Ciombor DM, et al. Perfusion abnormalities in subchondral bone associated with marrow edema, osteoarthritis, and avascular necrosis. Ann N Y Acad Sci 2007;1117:124–37; with permission.)

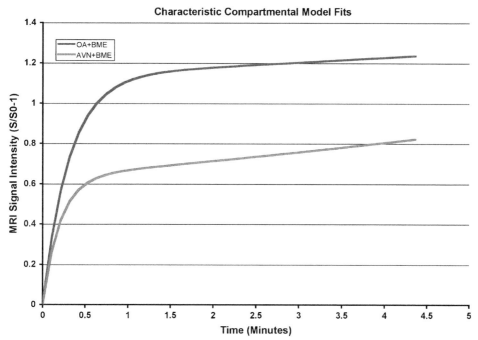

Fig. 4. Time intensity curves of a population of patients with abnormal edema separated by type of pathology (either AVN or OA). Slope and k_{el} are similar for both pathologies, but the amplitude is much less in AVN as compared with OA.

pressure and decreases in oxygen concentrations are seen in AVN and OA.[8] These studies were conducted with direct measurements in animals and humans and are invasive and technically difficult to perform. DCE-MRI is capable of extracting similar values using noninvasive methods.

Although initial observations of hypercoagulability were made in AVN, hypercoagulability also has been described in many patients who have OA.[1,2] Clinical studies have demonstrated that patients with end-stage hip arthritis exhibit a high

prevalence of vascular-related comorbidities, including ischemic heart disease and myocardial infarction and arterial and venous thrombi, including ischemic peripheral vascular disease and deep venous thrombosis.[22] Data from our group also suggested an increased prevalence of thrombotic disease in patients who have OA of the hip.[1]

In our results presented in this article, we observed differences in perfusion parameters in OA and AVN. Bone marrow lesions can arise from

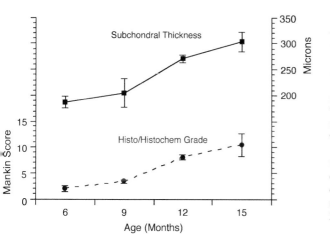

Fig. 5. Progression of cartilage and bone abnormalities in the Dunkin-Hartley guinea pig model of OA. The Mankin score at 9 months was 3.3 ± 0.33 compared with 8.0 ± 0.48 at 12 months (P < .001). Significant increases in medial tibial subchondral bone plate thickness are also observed between 9 and 12 months of age. The thickness at 9 months was 205 ± 27.66 μm compared with 270 ± 7.32 μm at 12 months (P = .003). (*From* Aaron RK, Dyke JP, Ciombor DM, et al. Perfusion abnormalities in subchondral bone associated with marrow edema, osteoarthritis, and avascular necrosis. Ann N Y Acad Sci 2007;1117:124–37; with permission.)

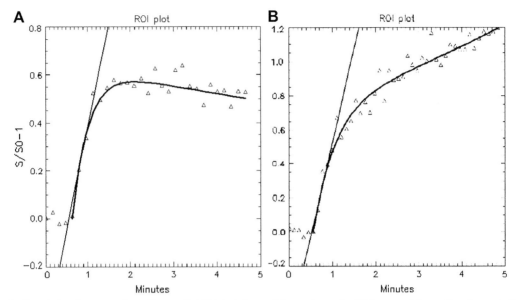

Fig. 6. Time intensity curves from the medial tibial plateau of the guinea pig. (*A*) Image at 6 months of age, before morphologic changes of OA, demonstrates normal perfusion with k_{el} = 0.06. (*B*) Twelve-month-old animals with established changes of OA revealed diminished perfusion with k_{el} = −0.11. (*From* Aaron RK, Dyke JP, Ciombor DM, et al. Perfusion abnormalities in subchondral bone associated with marrow edema, osteoarthritis, and avascular necrosis. Ann N Y Acad Sci 2007;1117:124–37; with permission.)

trauma and OA and AVN and may manifest as differences in pathophysiology and vascularity. Changes observed via DCE-MRI may be produced because of a combination of variances in capillary permeability and tissue perfusion and flow. Although the specific mechanisms of action are still being isolated, overall clearance of the contrast agent seems to be decreased in clinical and animal populations. The ability to image perfusion in bone safely and noninvasively is a powerful tool that can be used to diagnose and classify disorders of bone, not only those limited to OA and AVN.

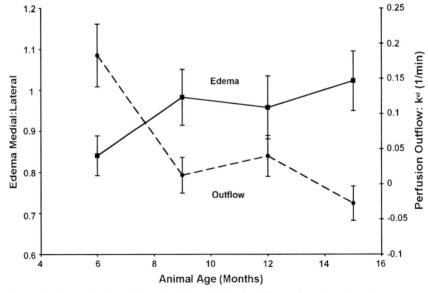

Fig. 7. Estimation of edema of the subchondral bone is derived from short tau inversion recovery images of regions of interest at the medial tibial plateau and adjacent lateral plateau and is expressed as voxel intensity ratio of medial:lateral trabecular bone. Edema of the medial:lateral tibial plateau increased between 6 and 9 months of age but did not reach statistical significance (P = .06).

REFERENCES

1. Aaron RK, Ciombor DM. Pain in osteoarthritis. Med Health R I 2004;87(7):205–9.
2. Cheras PA, Freemont AJ, Sikorski JM, et al. Intraosseous thrombosis in ischemic necrosis of bone and osteoarthritis. Osteoarthr Cartil 1993;1(4):219–32.
3. Okubo M, Kinoshita T, Yukimura T, et al. Experimental study of measurement of regional bone blood flow in the adult mongrel dog using radioactive microspheres. Clin Orthop Relat Res 1979;(138):263–70.
4. Felson DT, Chaisson CE, Hill CL, et al. The association of bone marrow lesions with pain in knee osteoarthritis. Ann Intern Med 2001;134(7):541–9.
5. Zanetti M, Bruder E, Romero J, et al. Bone marrow edema pattern in osteoarthritic knees: correlation between MR imaging and histologic findings. Radiology 2000;215(3):835–40.
6. Arnoldi CC. Vascular aspects of degenerative joint disorders: a synthesis. Acta Orthop Scand Suppl 1994;261:1–82.
7. Arnoldi CC, Lemperg K, Linderholm H, et al. Intraosseous hypertension and pain in the knee. J Bone Joint Surg Br 1975;57(3):360–3.
8. Arnoldi CC, Linderholm H, Mussbichler H, et al. Venous engorgement and intraosseous hypertension in osteoarthritis of the hip. J Bone Joint Surg Br 1972;54(3):409–21.
9. Lee JH, Dyke JP, Ballon D, et al. Subchondral fluid dynamics in a model of osteoarthritis: use of dynamic contrast-enhanced magnetic resonance imaging. Osteoarthr Cartil 2008; [Submitted].
10. Hoffmann U, Brix G, Knopp MV, et al. Pharmacokinetic mapping of the breast: a new method for dynamic MR mammography. Magn Reson Med 1995;33(4):506–14.
11. Brix G, Semmler W, Port R, et al. Pharmacokinetic parameters in CNS Gd-DTPA enhanced MR imaging. J Comput Assist Tomogr 1991;15(4):621–8.
12. Dyke JP, Panicek DM, Healey JH, et al. Osteogenic and Ewing sarcomas: estimation of necrotic fraction during induction chemotherapy with dynamic contrast-enhanced MR imaging. Radiology 2003; 228(1):271–8.
13. Bendele AM, Hulman JF. Spontaneous cartilage degeneration in guinea pigs. Arthritis Rheum 1988; 31(4):561–5.
14. Jimenez PA, Glasson SS, Trubetskoy OV, et al. Spontaneous osteoarthritis in Dunkin Hartley guinea pigs: histologic, radiologic, and biochemical changes. Lab Anim Sci 1997;47(6):598–601.
15. Wei L, Svensson O, Hjerpe A, et al. Correlation of morphologic and biochemical changes in the natural history of spontaneous osteoarthrosis in guinea pigs. Arthritis Rheum 1997;40(11):2075–83.
16. Watson PJ, Hall LD, Carpenter TA, et al. A magnetic resonance imaging study of joint degeneration in the guinea pig knee. Agents Actions Suppl 1993;39: 261–5.
17. Mankin HJ, Dorfman H, Lippiello L, et al. Biochemical and metabolic abnormalities in articular cartilage from osteo-arthritic human hips. II. Correlation of morphology with biochemical and metabolic data. J Bone Joint Surg Am 1971;53(3):523–37.
18. Aaron RK, Dyke JP, Ciombor DM, et al. Perfusion abnormalities in subchondral bone associated with marrow edema, osteoarthritis, and avascular necrosis. Ann N Y Acad Sci 2007;1117:124–37.
19. Tsukamoto H, Kang YS, Jones LC, et al. Evaluation of marrow perfusion in the femoral head by dynamic magnetic resonance imaging: effect of venous occlusion in a dog model. Invest Radiol 1992; 27(4):275–81.
20. Kiaer T, Pedersen NW, Kristensen KD, et al. Intraosseous pressure and oxygen tension in avascular necrosis and osteoarthritis of the hip. J Bone Joint Surg Br 1990;72(6):1023–30.
21. Kiaer T, Gronlund J, Sorensen KH, et al. Subchondral pO2, pCO2, pressure, pH, and lactate in human osteoarthritis of the hip. Clin Orthop Relat Res 1988;(229):149–55.
22. Marks R, Allegrante JP. Comorbid disease profiles of adults with end-stage hip osteoarthritis. Med Sci Monit 2002;8(4):CR305–9.

Collapsed Subchondral Fatigue Fracture of the Femoral Head

Young-Kyun Lee, MD[a], Jeong Joon Yoo, MD[b], Kyung-Hoi Koo, MD[a], Kang Sup Yoon, MD[c], Byung Woo Min, MD[d], Hee Joong Kim, MD[b],*

KEYWORDS

• Subchondral fracture • Femoral head • Collapse

Subchondral stress fracture of the femoral head (SSFFH) is a rarely encountered condition. It occurs not only as an insufficiency-type stress fracture in elderly people or in renal transplant recipients,[1–10] but also as a fatigue-type stress fracture in healthy adults.[11,12] As in osteonecrosis of the femoral head, which has very similar clinical features and imaging findings,[1–6,13–15] collapse of the femoral head can occur in fatigue-type SSFFH.[11,12,16] It is well known that once collapse of the femoral head takes place in osteonecrosis of the femoral head, the hip joint deteriorates rapidly and an arthroplasty is eventually necessary in most cases.[17,18] However, little is known about the fate of collapsed fatigue-type SSFFH.

The authors hypothesized that the fate of collapsed fatigue-type SSFFH probably differ from that of collapsed osteonecrosis of the femoral head because they are similar but quite separate disease conditions. The authors expected a much better prognosis in collapsed subchondral stress fractures because they have an intact blood supply and healing potential. In this study, the authors retrospectively evaluated the clinical course of collapsed fatigue-type SSFFH in nine patients.

MATERIALS AND METHODS

Between November 1999 and August 2005, nine consecutive subjects (nine hips: five right, four left) with a collapsed fatigue-type SSFFH were treated (**Table 1**). All subjects were men who had a mean age of 23 years (range, 20–34 years) at the time of hip pain onset. Eight subjects were soldiers when the hip pain started during military drills, such as a basic training immediately after recruitment or while practicing martial arts. One subject was an office worker and his hip pain developed after carrying heavy materials for 2 weeks. All subjects were otherwise healthy, had no history of any associated disease, and were not taking any medication. All subjects participated in this study with informed consent, and the study protocol was approved by the Institutional Review Board of the authors' hospital.

A diagnosis of SSFFH was based on typical plain radiograph and MRI findings. In all cases, collapse of the femoral head was evident on plain radiographs. MRI findings of SSFFH included a subchondral low-signal intensity band on T1-weighted images (MR crescent sign), and surrounding bone marrow edema (**Fig. 1**).[1,3–5,7,9,19]

This work was supported by Grant No. 06-03-063 from the Seoul National University Hospital Research Fund.
[a] Department of Orthopaedic Surgery, Seoul National University Bundang Hospital, 300 Gumidong Bundanggu, Seongnam, 463-707, Korea
[b] Department of Orthopaedic Surgery, Seoul National University College of Medicine, Seoul National University Hospital, 28 Youngondong Chongnogu, Seoul, 110-744, Korea
[c] Department of Orthopaedic Surgery, Seoul Municipal Boramae Hospital, Seoul National University College of Medicine, 395 Shindaebangdong Dongjackgu, Seoul, 156-707, Korea
[d] Department of Orthopaedic Surgery, Keimyung University, School of Medicine, Dongsan Medical Center, 194 Dongsandong, Joonggu, Daegu, 700-712, Korea
* Corresponding author.
E-mail address: oskim@snu.ac.kr (H. Kim).

Orthop Clin N Am 40 (2009) 259–265
doi:10.1016/j.ocl.2008.10.008

Table 1
Demographic, clinical, and imaging findings of patients with subchondral fracture of the femoral head

Case	Age (Years)	Height (cm)/Weight (kg)	Job	Affected Side	Duration of Pain[a] (Months)	Follow-Up (Years)	Last Degree of Collapse	Latest K/L[b] Grade	Harris Hip Score	WOMAC[c]	UCLA[d]	Treatment
1	21	165/55	Military recruit	R	7	3.0	Moderate	0	93	10	3	Nonweight-bearing
2	34	170/65	Office worker	R	7	4.5	Mild	0	97	3	4	Nonweight-bearing
3	23	165/78	Soldier	L	9	6.3	Severe	2	97	3	5	Nonweight-bearing
4	22	172/60	Military recruit	L	8	5.4	Moderate	2	81	12	3	Nonweight-bearing
5	20	170/73	Military recruit	L	6	3.1	Mild	0	93	10	3	Nonweight-bearing
6	21	170/65	Military recruit	R	9	6.3	Moderate	0	93	7	5	Nonweight-bearing
7	21	190/80	Military recruit	R	7	6.3	Moderate	2	91	12	4	Impaction bone grafting
8	20	181/64	Military recruit	R	5	8.3	Mild	2	97	8	5	Multiple drilling
9	21	170/61	Soldier	L	5	9.0	Mild	2	81	12	3	Multiple drilling

[a] From onset to complete disappearance.
[b] Kellgren-Lawrence.
[c] Western Ontario and McMaster University Osteoarthritis Index.
[d] University of California at Los Angeles.

A

B

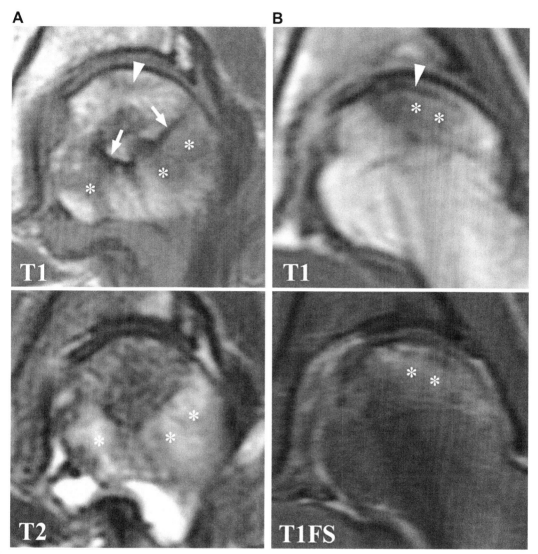

Fig. 1. (A) A typical case of osteonecrosis of the femoral head. The outer margin of the necrotic lesion is delineated as an abnormal signal intensity band (arrows, reactive margin) outside the subchondral fracture line (arrowhead). The bone marrow edema pattern (asterisks) is observed only outside the necrotic area. (B) A typical case of subchondral stress fracture of the femoral head. A subchondral fracture line (arrowhead) exists in the subchondral area, and the bone-marrow-edema pattern (asterisks) extends to the subchondral area. There is no additional abnormal signal intensity band representing the reactive margin of the necrotic area.

Eight of the nine subjects visited the authors' outpatient clinic more than 3 months after the onset of hip pain. All of them had been previously treated conservatively at other hospitals. Two of them, the earliest cases in this series, underwent multiple drilling under a misdiagnosis of osteonecrosis of the femoral head (ONFH). In these cases, the operation was performed when hip pain disappeared almost completely, and no change in femoral head contour was observed postoperatively. Six cases were treated conservatively by weight-bearing as

tolerated until the hip pain completely disappeared. The remaining subject, who presented 6 weeks after the onset of hip pain, was treated by impaction iliac bone grafting, which elevated the collapse but not completely (from grade C to grade B) (**Fig. 2**).

Follow-up radiographic and clinical examinations were performed every 1 to 2 months until complete hip pain disappearance, and annually thereafter. At the time of the study, six subjects were willing and able to return to the authors' clinic

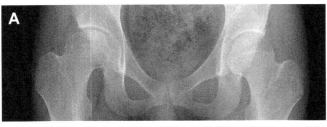

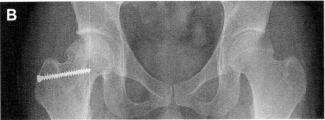

Fig. 2. A 21-year-old military recruit with a right subchondral fatigue fracture of the femoral head (Patient 7). (*A*) An anteroposterior radiograph obtained 1 month after right hip pain onset shows marked collapse in the right femoral head. (*B*) An anteroposterior radiograph obtained 6 years and 4 months after impaction bone grafting shows that the fracture healed with partial recovery of the collapse in the right femoral head. Tönnis grade 1 degenerative change is observed.

for full clinical and radiographic evaluations, but three subjects were not and completed telephone and postal questionnaires instead.

Clinical assessments were performed 3 to 9 years (mean, 5.8 years) after the onset of hip pain using Harris Hip Scores for clinical outcome, WOMAC scores for hip function, and UCLA scores for rating at current activity levels.[20–23]

On plain radiographs, maximum depression of the collapsed femoral heads were measured using concentric circles and cases were then graded according to the ARCO system:[24] Grade A, mild depression (<2 mm); Grade B, moderate depression (2 mm–4 mm); and Grade C, severe depression (>4 mm). Degenerative changes in affected hips were evaluated using the modified Tönnis grading system,[25–27] and the Kellgren-Lawrence Radiographic Grading Scale[28] on latest radiographs taken 3 to 8.8 years (mean, 5.2 years) after hip pain onset.

RESULTS

In all nine subjects, hip pain decreased gradually eventually disappeared completely, and there were no recurrences. Mean duration of hip pain was 7.2 months (range, 5–9 months). Follow-up MRI obtained for seven subjects showed gradual disappearance of bone marrow edema and subchondral fracture lines. At latest follow-up, mean Harris Hip Score was 91.4 points (range, 81–97), mean WOMAC score was 8.6 points (range, 3–12), and UCLA scales ranged from 3 to 5 (median, 4) (see **Table 1**). No subject had a limitation of daily activity and all subjects participated in light sports activities.

In all cases, the anterosuperior portion of the femoral head had collapsed. Average maximum depression measured on radiographs taken after complete disappearance of hip pain was 2.8 mm (range, 0.9 mm–6.8 mm). There were four cases of grade A (mild, <2-mm depression), four cases

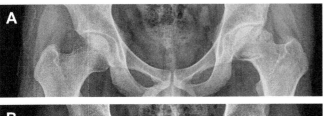

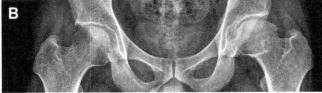

Fig. 3. A 23-year-old military soldier with a left subchondral fatigue fracture of the femoral head (Patient 3). (*A*) An anteroposterior radiograph obtained 5 months after left hip pain onset shows severe collapse in the left femoral head. (*B*) An anteroposterior radiograph obtained 6 years and 4 months after hip pain onset shows that the degree of collapse in the left femoral head did not progress. Tönnis grade 1 degenerative change is observed.

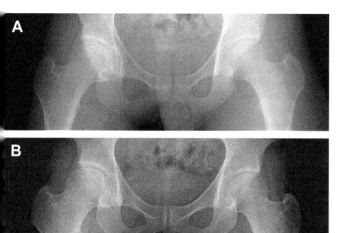

Fig. 4. A 21-year-old military soldier with a right subchondral fatigue fracture of the femoral head (Patient 6). (*A*) An anteroposterior radiograph obtained 4 months after right hip pain onset shows moderate collapse in the right femoral head. (*B*) An anteroposterior radiograph obtained 6 years and 2 months after hip pain onset shows that the degree of collapse did not progress in the right femoral head. No degenerative change is observed.

of grade B (moderate, 2-mm to 4-mm depression), and one case of grade C (severe, >4-mm depression). Compared with initial radiographs, no significant progression of the depression was detected on follow-up radiographs in all cases except one case, in which the collapsed portion was partially elevated by impaction iliac bone grafting. On latest radiographs, no progression of femoral head collapse was detected. In five hips (two cases of grade A, two cases of grade B, and one case of grade C depression), degenerative change of Tönnis grade 1 and Kellgren-Lawrence Scale 2 was observed (**Fig. 3**). No degenerative change was detected in the remaining four hips (two cases of grade A, two cases of grade B) (**Fig. 4**).

Table 2
Literature review

Authors	No. of Patients (No. of Cases)	Mean Age (Range)	Sex (M/F)	Type of Stress Fracture
Bangil et al[1]	2 (2)	74 (72–76)	0/2	Insufficiency
Rafii et al[3]	3 (4)	68 (63–76)	1/2	Insufficiency
Hagino et al[9]	2 (2)	75 (74–75)	0/2	Insufficiency
Yamamoto et al[4]	10 (10)	75 (65–88)	0/10	Insufficiency
Yamamoto et al[5]	1 (1)	65	0/1	Insufficiency
Yamamoto et al[8]	11 (11)	69 (61–78)	2/9	Insufficiency
Yamamoto et al[7]	1 (1)	69	1/0	Insufficiency
Yamamoto et al[6]	7 (7)	72 (65–81)	1/6	Insufficiency
Motomura et al[14]	1 (1)	64	0/1	Insufficiency
Buttaro et al[2]	4 (4)	70 (68–74)	0/4	Insufficiency
Uetani et al[15]	1 (1)	76	0/1	Insufficiency
Song et al[11]	5 (7)	21 (20–22)	5/0	Fatigue
Huang et al[32]	1 (1)	31	0/1	Insufficiency
Niimi et al[33]	1 (1)	75	0/1	Insufficiency
Ikemura et al[10]	1 (2)	47	1/0	Insufficiency
Chan et al[31]	1 (2)	65	0/1	Insufficiency
Kim et al[12]	4 (5)	39 (33–46)	3/1	Fatigue
Present Study	9 (9)	23 (20–34)	9/0	Fatigue

Abbreviations: M, male; F, female.

Table 3
Distinguishing features of osteonecrosis of the femoral head and subchondral stress fracture of the femoral head

	ONFH	SSFFH
Incidence	15,000 cases per year in the United States[17,24]	Rare
Predisposing factors	Alcohol, high-dose corticosteroid, idiopathic, posttraumatic, organ transplantation, sickle cell disease, Gaucher disease, and others.	Fatigue type: recent increase in activity; Insufficiency type: osteoporosis
Laterality	Bilateral in more than 50% of patients	Unknown
Progression	Usually progress to end-stage degenerative joint disease	Benign course according to current study
MRI findings	Subchondral fracture; Reactive margin (outer margin of the necrotic lesion, low signal band on T1);[35,36] Bone marrow edema outside the necrotic area	Subchondral fracture; No reactive margin; Bone marrow edema up to the fracture line

DISCUSSION

It has been reported that collapse of the femoral head occurs in fatigue-type SSFFH.[11,12,29] However, most reported cases of collapsed SSFFH were insufficiency-type fractures and have been treated by total hip arthroplasty (**Table 2**).[1–10,14,15,30–33] The reasons for surgery included intractable pain and misdiagnosis as a collapsed ONFH. There is a possibility that more severe collapse occurs in insufficiency-type fractures than in fatigue-type fractures because of poor bone quality, and Yamamoto and colleagues[8] reported that insufficiency-type SSFFH might lead to rapid hip destruction. In contrast, as shown in the present study, collapse of the femoral head in fatigue-type SSFFH is not progressive and the pain disappears gradually. These observations suggest that conservative treatment with protected weight-bearing or impaction bone grafting can be attempted in collapsed insufficiency-type SSFFH before performing total hip arthroplasty.

All subjects enrolled in this study were informed that early degenerative changes would occur in their affected hip joints because of the deformed natures of the femoral heads, especially if the joint was exposed to heavy loading. In the present study, two subjects did not attempt any sports activity, even a light one, even though they were feeling that they could. This seems to be the reason for the relatively low UCLA scores. In five out of nine subjects, mild-degenerative change was observed on latest radiographs, but its existence did not correlate with the Harris Hip Scores or WOMAC scores.

Because subchondral fracture and bone marrow edema also occur commonly in ONFH, SSFFH can be misdiagnosed as ONFH.[8,12,34] In the present study, two early cases were misdiagnosed as ONFH initially and were surgically treated in accordance with ONFH. Once subchondral collapse occurs in ONFH, both clinical symptoms and radiologic collapse are usually progressive,[17,18] and subsequent degenerative changes finally progress to joint destruction. In contrast, the present study demonstrates that collapsed fatigue-type SSFFH heals without progression of the collapse or joint destruction and clinical symptoms disappear (**Table 3**).

Despite the small number of subjects enrolled in the present study, collapsed fatigue-type SSFFH showed a benign clinical course, unlike collapsed ONFH.

REFERENCES

1. Bangil M, Soubrier M, Dubost JJ, et al. Subchondral insufficiency fracture of the femoral head. Rev Rhum Engl Ed 1996;63(11):859–61.
2. Buttaro M, Della Valle AG, Morandi A, et al. Insufficiency subchondral fracture of the femoral head: report of 4 cases and review of the literature. J Arthroplasty 2003;18(3):377–82.
3. Rafii M, Mitnick H, Klug J, et al. Insufficiency fracture of the femoral head: MR imaging in three patients. AJR Am J Roentgenol 1997;168(1):159–63.
4. Yamamoto T, Bullough PG. Subchondral insufficiency fracture of the femoral head: a differential

diagnosis in acute onset of coxarthrosis in the elderly. Arthritis Rheum 1999;42(12):2719–23.

5. Yamamoto T, Schneider R, Bullough PG. Insufficiency subchondral fracture of the femoral head. Am J Surg Pathol 2000;24(3):464–8.

6. Yamamoto T, Schneider R, Bullough PG. Subchondral insufficiency fracture of the femoral head: histopathologic correlation with MRI. Skeletal Radiol 2001;30(5):247–54.

7. Yamamoto T, Bullough PG. Subchondral insufficiency fracture of the femoral head and medial femoral condyle. Skeletal Radiol 2000;29(1):40–4.

8. Yamamoto T, Bullough PG. The role of subchondral insufficiency fracture in rapid destruction of the hip joint: a preliminary report. Arthritis Rheum 2000; 43(11):2423–7.

9. Hagino H, Okano T, Teshima R, et al. Insufficiency fracture of the femoral head in patients with severe osteoporosis—report of 2 cases. Acta Orthop Scand 1999;70(1):87–9.

10. Ikemura S, Yamamoto T, Nakashima Y, et al. Bilateral subchondral insufficiency fracture of the femoral head after renal transplantation: a case report. Arthritis Rheum 2005;52(4):1293–6.

11. Song WS, Yoo JJ, Koo KH, et al. Subchondral fatigue fracture of the femoral head in military recruits. J Bone Joint Surg Am 2004;86-A(9):1917–24.

12. Kim JW, Yoo JJ, Min BW, et al. Subchondral fracture of the femoral head in healthy adults. Clin Orthop Relat Res 2007;464:196–204.

13. Todd RC, Freeman MA, Pirie CJ. Isolated trabecular fatigue fractures in the femoral head. J Bone Joint Surg Br 1972;54(4):723–8.

14. Motomura G, Yamamoto T, Miyanishi K, et al. Subchondral insufficiency fracture of the femoral head and acetabulum: a case report. J Bone Joint Surg Am 2002;84-A(7):1205–9.

15. Uetani M, Hashmi R, Ito M, et al. Subchondral insufficiency fracture of the femoral head: magnetic resonance imaging findings correlated with microcomputed tomography and histopathology. J Comput Assist Tomogr 2003;27(2):189–93.

16. Freeman MA, Day WH, Swanson SA. Fatigue fracture in the subchondral bone of the human cadaver femoral head. Med Biol Eng 1971;9(6):619–29.

17. Guerra JJ, Steinberg ME. Distinguishing transient osteoporosis from avascular necrosis of the hip. J Bone Joint Surg Am 1995;77(4):616–24.

18. Mankin HJ. Nontraumatic necrosis of bone (osteonecrosis). N Engl J Med 1992;326(22):1473–9.

19. Vande Berg BC, Malghem J, Goffin EJ, et al. Transient epiphyseal lesions in renal transplant recipients: presumed insufficiency stress fractures. Radiology 1994;191(2):403–7.

20. Harris WH. Traumatic arthritis of the hip after dislocation and acetabular fractures: treatment by mold arthroplasty. An end-result study using a new method of result evaluation. J Bone Joint Surg Am 1969;51(4):737–55.

21. Amstutz HC, Thomas BJ, Jinnah R, et al. Treatment of primary osteoarthritis of the hip. A comparison of total joint and surface replacement arthroplasty. J Bone Joint Surg Am 1984;66(2):228–41.

22. Zahiri CA, Schmalzried TP, Szuszczewicz ES, et al. Assessing activity in joint replacement patients. J Arthroplasty 1998;13(8):890–5.

23. Bellamy N, Buchanan WW, Goldsmith CH, et al. Validation study of WOMAC: a health status instrument for measuring clinically important patient relevant outcomes to antirheumatic drug therapy in patients with osteoarthritis of the hip or knee. J Rheumatol 1988;15(12):1833–40.

24. Mont MA, Hungerford DS. Non-traumatic avascular necrosis of the femoral head. J Bone Joint Surg Am 1995;77(3):459–74.

25. Millis MB, Murphy SB. Use of computed tomographic reconstruction in planning osteotomies of the hip. Clin Orthop Relat Res 1992;274:154–9.

26. Tonnis D, Behrens K, Tscharani F. A modified technique of the triple pelvic osteotomy: early results. J Pediatr Orthop 1981;1(3):241–9.

27. Tonnis D. An evaluation of conservative and operative methods in the treatment of congenital hip dislocation. Clin Orthop Relat Res 1976;119:76–88.

28. Kellgren JH, Lawrence JS. Radiological assessment of osteo-arthrosis. Ann Rheum Dis 1957;16(4):494–502.

29. Visuri T. Stress osteopathy of the femoral head. 10 military recruits followed for 5–11 years. Acta Orthop Scand 1997;68(2):138–41.

30. Yamamoto T, Kubo T, Hirasawa Y, et al. A clinicopathologic study of transient osteoporosis of the hip. Skeletal Radiol 1999;28(11):621–7.

31. Chan CC, Li A, Fan WC, et al. Subchondral insufficiency fracture of the femoral head. Hong Kong Med J 2006;12(6):460–2.

32. Huang KC, Hsu WH, Lee KF, et al. Subchondral insufficiency fracture with rapid collapse of the femoral head in a patient with Turner's syndrome. Rheumatology (Oxford) 2005;44(6):826–7.

33. Niimi R, Hasegawa M, Sudo A, et al. Rapidly destructive coxopathy after subchondral insufficiency fracture of the femoral head. Arch Orthop Trauma Surg 2005;125(6):410–3.

34. Aigner N, Schneider W, Eberl V, et al. Core decompression in early stages of femoral head osteonecrosis—an MRI-controlled study. Int Orthop 2002;26(1):31–5.

35. Mitchell DG, Steinberg ME, Dalinka MK, et al. Magnetic resonance imaging of the ischemic hip. Alterations within the osteonecrotic, viable, and reactive zones. Clin Orthop Relat Res 1989;244:60–77.

36. Glimcher MJ, Kenzora JE. Nicolas Andry Award. The biology of osteonecrosis of the human femoral head and its clinical implications: 1. Tissue biology. Clin Orthop Relat Res 1979;138:284–309.

Respherical Contour with Medial Collapsed Femoral Head Necrosis After High-Degree Posterior Rotational Osteotomy in Young Patients with Extensive Necrosis

Takashi Atsumi, MD, PhD*, Toshihisa Kajiwara, MD, PhD,
Satoshi Tamaoki, MD, PhD, Akihiko Maeda, MD, PhD,
Ryo Nakanishi, MD, PhD

KEYWORDS

- Osteonecrosis • Femoral head necrosis
- Osteotomy • Collapse • Subchondral fracture

Osteonecrosis of the femoral head often occurs in patients under the age of 50 years. If the necrotic focus is small and located out of the loaded portion of the femoral head, collapse is not likely to develop.[1] If the necrotic focus is predominantly located in the superolateral loaded portion of the femoral head, however, it results in progressive collapse,[2] and generally the joint is affected by secondary osteoarthritis and undergoes prosthetic replacement.[3–7] The results of prosthetic replacement for young patients with osteonecrosis, however, are often not optimal.[3–5] The authors believe that preservation of the affected joint is important in young patients to avoid joint-replacement procedures. The joint-preserving procedures are usually effective for hips with small- or medium-sized lesions in early stage of the disease.[8–11] In advanced stage with extensive collapsed lesions, any kind of treatment approaches for preservation of the joint[9–11] are usually not effective. When patients with extensive necrotic esions visit the hospital for the first time, collapse has already taken place in many cases.

Transtrochanteric anterior rotational osteotomy developed by Sugioka and coworkers[12] for osteonecrosis of the femoral head with extensive lesion is an ideal treatment even for patients with evidence of collapse. Although Sugioka[13] mentioned the possibility of posterior rotational osteotomy, he did not report on the results in detail. The authors have previously reported on the use of posterior rotational osteotomies including a modified approach, high-degree posterior rotational osteotomy,[14–17] for femoral head osteonecrosis with extensive lesions and progressive collapse. By means of high posterior rotational osteotomy for markedly collapsed cases, uncollapsed anterior viable areas are transferred to the loaded portion below the acetabular roof, and the collapsed necrotic focus is moved to the medial portion of the femoral head, which can be confirmed on postoperative anteroposterior radiographs (**Fig. 1**).[17] In

Department of Orthopaedic Surgery, Showa University Fujigaoka Hospital, Showa University School of Medicine, 1–30 Fujigaoka Aobaku, Yokohama 227-8501, Japan
* Corresponding author.
E-mail address: t.atsumi@showa-university-fujigaoka.gr.jp (T. Atsumi).

Orthop Clin N Am 40 (2009) 267–274
doi:10.1016/j.ocl.2008.10.012
0030-5898/08/$ – see front matter © 2009 Elsevier Inc. All rights reserved.

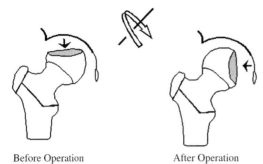

Before Operation   After Operation

Fig. 1. Schematic. A high-degree posterior rotational osteotomy for femoral head osteonecrosis with extensive collapsed lesion. Before the operation, the apparent collapsed necrotic lesion (*arrow*) is extended laterally to the acetabular edge without viable area on loaded portion below the acetabulum. After the operation, the collapsed necrotic area is moved medially (*arrow*) on the anteroposterior radiograph.

this study, the authors evaluated the effectiveness of high-degree posterior rotation in terms of regaining the spherical contour of severely collapsed necrotic femoral head that was moved medially, and they also investigated whether or not subchondral fracture disappeared on the medial femoral head on postoperative anteroposterior radiographs as a result of remodeling after this procedure.

MATERIALS AND METHODS

Between the end of 1985 and the beginning of 2002, posterior rotational osteotomies including high-degree posterior rotation developed by Atsumi and coworkers[14–17] were performed on 48 hips of young patients (<50 years of age), who were affected by nontraumatic or traumatic osteonecrosis of the femoral head. Of these hips, 28 hips in 24 patients were reviewed at a minimum of 5-year follow-up (range, 5–14 years; mean, 8.5 years). Twenty seven of 28 hips were not converted to a prosthetic replacement because most patients had minimal or no pain. One hip was converted to a prosthetic replacement because of severe pain, and follow-up ended at that time.

In these 28 hips, preoperative collapsed areas were moved to the medial portion, and collapsed areas were clearly observed at the medial portion of the femoral head during the short period after surgery on postoperative anteroposterior radiographs (**Figs. 2**A and **3**A). Postoperative anteroposterior radiographs of these 28 hips at 6 months, at 3 years, and at final follow-up were observed. Analysis was made radiographically, which initially demonstrated collapse of the femoral head after surgery and observed how spherical contour was regained or not in the collapsed area

that was moved to medial portion. Twenty of 48 hips were excluded from the study; 11 hips regained a spherical contour in the necrotic lesion of the medial femoral head immediately after surgery on anteroposterior radiographs (because the objective is to evaluate the process of remodeling, the focus was only on the hips, which initially had collapse on the femoral head after surgery, and tried to observe how the collapsed area improves); four hips were lost to follow-up; two hips were converted to prosthetic replacement at less than 5 years after surgery because of early recollapse; one patient died of underlying disease; one hip had a deep infection; and one hip had the onset of rheumatoid arthritis.

In the evaluable 28 hips, the age of the patients at the time of surgery ranged from 15 to 49 years with a mean of 26 years. Nine patients were women and 15 were men. A total of 22 hips were nontraumatic, and 6 were traumatic. Sixteen hips in 12 patients had a history of corticosteroid administration. The underlying diseases of these 12 patients were systemic lupus erythematosus in three patients, nephrosis in two patients, bronchial asthma in two patients, aplastic anemia in one patient, multiple sclerosis in one patient, pemphigus vulgaris in one patient, hepatitis in one patient, and brain injury in one patient. In the remaining 12 hips in 12 patients, six hips in six patients had apparent alcohol abuse, and six hips in six patients were traumatic (following neck fracture, five hips; traumatic posterior dislocation, one hip).

All 28 hips had extensive lesions from medial to lateral and from anterior to the posterior portion of the femoral head with no viable area on the articular surface of the weight-bearing portion of the femoral head facing the acetabular roof on preoperative anteroposterior radiographs (**Figs. 2**B and **3**B) (type C2 according to the criteria of the Japanese Investigations Committee [see **Fig. 1**]).[18] Apparent collapse was noted in all hips preoperatively. Degree of collapse was greater than 3 mm in all hips (see **Fig. 1**), and no apparent joint space narrowing was noted in 23 of 28 hips (stage 3B based on the criteria of the Japanese Investigations Committee) (**Fig. 3**C).[18] The remaining five hips, however, showed apparent joint space narrowing (**Fig. 2**C). According to the Association Research Circulation Osseous classification,[19] 23 hips showed stage III with type C location, and stage IV in five hips. The necrotic lesion extended from the anterior to posterior portion in all hips. On lateral radiographs,[13] the posterior viable area of the joint surface of these hips before surgery ranged from 6% to 25% (mean, 15%). The anterior viable area ranged from 7% to 41% (mean, 19%).[17] All hips were out of indication for a traditional anterior rotational

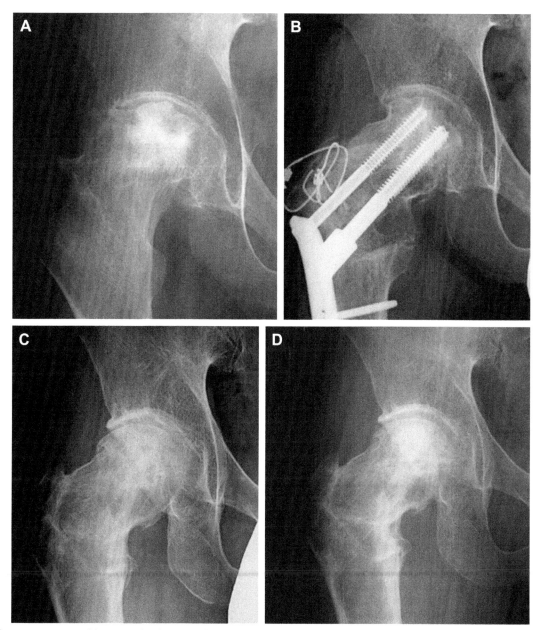

Fig. 2. A 20-year-old man with a history of aplastic anemia treated with high dose of corticosteroids. (*A*) A preoperative anteroposterior radiograph of his right hip showed severe collapsed lesion with joint space narrowing. (*B*) An anteroposterior radiograph 3 months after 135-degree posterior rotation with 15-degree varus position. The viable area was noted on the superior femoral head, although the shape was still erratic. Note the collapsed lesion was moved medially. (*C*) An anteroposterior radiograph taken 3 years after operation showed resphericity of medial femoral head shape. Note the extended joint space and improved shape of acetabular subchondral roof. (*D*) An anteroposterior radiograph taken 14 years after operation disclosed spherical contour of the medial femoral head and maintenance of joint space.

osteotomy. Sixteen cases were bilaterally affected by nontraumatic osteonecrosis as determined by radiographs or MRI. Of these cases, nine cases were treated by bilateral high-degree posterior rotational osteotomy. Different procedures were elected for the contralateral hips of the other three nontraumatic cases: one anterior rotational osteotomy, one femoral varus osteotomy, and one total hip arthroplasty. The remaining four were not treated because the necrotic lesion was

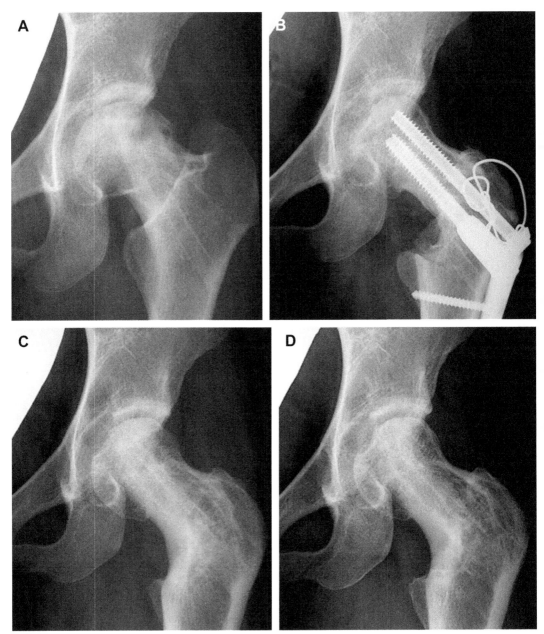

Fig. 3. A 22-year-old woman with traumatic femoral head necrosis following left femoral neck fracture. (*A*) She received open reduction and internal fixation using cancellous screws at another hospital. A preoperative anteroposterior radiograph of her left hip 1 year and 6 months after trauma showed a large collapsed lesion. (*B*) A 110-degree posterior rotational osteotomy with 10-degree varus position was performed. An anteroposterior radiograph taken 3 months after the operation revealed adequate viable joint surface of the femoral head below the acetabular roof. Note the necrotic collapsed lesion is moved to the medial area. (*C*) An anteroposterior radiograph taken 3 years after the operation disclosed spherical contour of the medial femoral head. The acetabular subchondral roof was also well remodeled. (*D*) An anteroposterior radiograph taken 7 years after the operation disclosed spherical contour of the medial femoral head and maintenance of joint space.

small in size without symptoms. In six traumatic cases, the contralateral hips were normal, and treatment was not performed. These hips were not included in this study.

The degree of posterior rotation ranged from 110 to 150 degrees posteriorly with a mean of 135 degrees. Ten to 25 degrees (mean, 18 degrees) of intentional varus positioning was affected in addition to the rotation in all 28 hips to obtain an extensive noncollapsed viable articular surface of the femoral head in loaded portion postoperatively. A summary of the patient population is shown in **Box 1**.

For the surgical procedure of posterior rotational osteotomy, a modified Southern approach[14,20] with patients placed in lateral position was used in all 28 hips. The skin incision passed 1 cm anteriorly from anterior margin of the greater trochanter for exposure of the anterior joint. The hip was rotated internally. The short external rotators, the obturator externus, and the iliopsoas tendon were incised with protection of the nutrient vessels. After an osteotomy of the greater trochanter,

the joint capsule was exposed, and circumferential incision of capsule was performed to achieve adequate rotation without vascular impairment. To determine the correct osteotomy plane, maximum length of neck was confirmed with the hip in internal rotation using fluoroscopy.

One K-wire was inserted to the center line of the femoral neck from the osteotomized area of greater trochanter for decision of axis of the femoral neck, followed by insertion of two K-wires into the femoral neck, which should meet the perpendicular axis of the femoral neck to determine the correct osteotomy plane. The osteotomy was performed by a reciprocating saw. For the fixation of osteotomy plane after femoral head rotation, an AO plate was used on one hip. A fixation device designed by Atsumi was used in the remaining 27 hips for strong fixation to allow for early range-of-motion exercise.

For postoperative management, early motion exercise and isometric exercise of quadriceps were started after the patients tolerated postoperative pain. The patients were in bed for 1 or 2 weeks depending on degree of posterior rotation and then used a wheelchair. Partial weight-bearing was started 5 to 6 weeks after operation using two crutches. Gait with one crutch was essential for 6 months to 1 year depending on the size of lesion because subchondral bone of the femoral head at the loaded portion moved by rotation had a weakness to weight-bearing during the early period after operation.

Mean postoperative viable area below the acetabular roof was measured by the method of Atsumi and Kuroki.[14] In all 28 hips, the degree of spherical contour regained in the collapsed femoral head, which was moved medially, was analyzed on postoperative anteroposterior radiographs at less than 6 months, at 3 years, and at final follow up. Measurements were performed where there was the greatest collapse of the medial femoral head on the postoperative anteroposterior radiographs. The outline of a normal femoral head was drawn, and a normal contour without collapse was determined.[7] The distance A (millimeter) was measured from hip center to superior viable joint surface. The distance B (millimeter) was also measured from a normal contour of the femoral head to medial area with the greatest collapse. The ratio of depth of collapse at medial collapsed femoral head was determined by B/A (percent) (**Fig. 4**).

The clinical condition was evaluated in points of pain, walking, and range-of-motion by modified Merle d'Aubigne hip scores described by Moed and colleagues.[21] Eighteen points was considered excellent, 17 very good, 15 to 16 good, 13 or 14 fair, and less than 13 poor.

Box 1
Summary of patient population with extensive collapsed necrotic lesion subjected in this study

Summary of patient population

28 hips of 24 patients with extensive or collapsed femoral head osteonecrosis.

Age: 15–49 years old (mean, 26 years).

Gender: 9 women, 15 men.

Etiologic factor

Steroid administration, 16 hips; alcohol abuse, 6 hips; trauma, 6 hips.

Extent of necrotic lesion

Anteroposterior radiographs.

Extensive lesions from medial to lateral and from anterior to the posterior portion of the femoral head with no viable area on loaded portion facing the acetabular roof (type C2 on criteria of the Japanese Investigations Committee).

Lateral radiographs

Anterior viable area, 7%–41% (mean, 19); posterior viable area, 6%–25% (mean, 15).

Stage

Stage 3B, 23 hips; stage 4, five hips on criteria of the Japanese Investigations Committee.

Stage II, 23 hips; stage IV, five hips on the Association Research Circulation Osseous classification.

Degree of collapse: greater than 3 mm in 28 hips on anteroposterior radiographs

Posterior rotational angle: 110–150 degrees (mean, 135 degrees)

Additional varus position: 10–25 degrees (mean, 18 degrees)

Follow-up: 5–14 years (mean, 8.5 years)

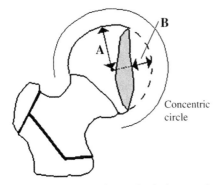

Fig. 4. Diagram showing the method of measuring the ratio of depth of collapse at medial collapsed femoral head after operation. Measurement was performed that showed the greatest collapse area of the medial femoral head on the postoperative anteroposterior radiographs. The shape of the outline of the femoral head is drawn, and a normal contour without collapse is determined. The distance A (millimeter) is measured from hip center to superior viable joint surface. The distance B (millimeter) is also measured from drawing out the line of normal contour of the femoral head to medial area of greatest collapse. The ratio of depth of collapse at medial collapsed femoral head was determined as B/A (%).

RESULTS

Anterior viable areas of the affected femoral heads were transferred to the loaded portion below the acetabular roof in all 28 hips. The mean postoperative viable area below the acetabular roof was from 28% to 100% with a mean of 58% on anteroposterior radiographs at less than 6 months after operation. All 28 hips were prevented from collapse of the loaded portion below the acetabular roof without evidence of osteonecrotic cysts in the weight-bearing portion on final anteroposterior radiographs. A total of 26 hips showed the maintenance of joint space. Slight progressive joint space narrowing was found in the remaining two hips. In five hips with apparent joint space narrowing preoperatively, the joint space was increased when compared with before the procedure, and maintained at final follow-up anteroposterior radiographs.

The collapsed necrotic area was observed in the medial portion on anteroposterior radiographs of all hips at less than 6 months, at 3 years, and at final follow-up postoperatively.

The degree of regaining of spherical contour of all 28 hips, which is represented by the ratio of medial collapse of the femoral head, was 5% to 45% (mean, 18.4%; standard deviation [SD], 9.4) less than 6 months after operation. Three years after surgery, the degree of collapse declined to 0% to 22% (mean, 8.3%; SD, 6.6) and down to 0% to

14% (mean, 3.4%; SD, 3.7) at final follow-up (5–14 years; mean, 8.5 years) (see **Figs. 2** and **3**; **Fig. 5**).

In 22 hips with nontraumatic necrosis, the mean ratio of respherical contour was 17.9% (SD, 9.2; range, 5–45) less than 6 months after operation; 8.4% (SD, 6.8; range, 0–22) 3 years after surgery; and 3.4% (SD, 3.2; range, 0–14) at final follow-up (**Fig. 2**D). On six hips of traumatic cases, the mean ratio of respherical contour was 20.3% (SD, 7.8; range, 13–30) less than 6 months after operation; 8% (SD, 4.3; range, 4–16) 3 years after surgery; and 3.3% (SD, 1.8; range, 0–5) at final follow-up (**Fig. 3**D).

Subchondral fracture of postoperative medial femoral head was clearly seen in 25 of 28 hips less than 6 months after surgery. Subchondral fracture disappeared on 17 hips (68%) 3 years after surgery, and on 23 hips (92%) at final follow-up (see **Fig. 3**). Of the remaining two hips, recollapse did not occur, although subchondral fracture was seen on final postoperative radiographs. In three of the hips for which subchondral fracture was not seen less than 6 months after surgery, recollapse was not observed on final postoperative radiographs with respherical contour with medial collapsed femoral head.

In 20 hips of nontraumatic necrosis, subchondral fracture disappeared in 15 hips (75%) 3 years after surgery, and 18 hips (90%) at final follow-up. In five hips with traumatic necrosis, subchondral fracture disappeared on two hips (40%) 3 years after surgery, and on five hips (100%) at final follow-up.

Clinically, pain at final follow-up included 23 of 28 hips with no pain with normal activity. Mild and inconstant pain occurred in five hips. Of these five hips, two hips showed joint space narrowing. The mean flexion angle was 105 degrees (range,

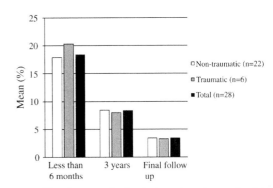

Fig. 5. The degree of spherical contour is regained in the postoperative medial collapsed femoral head, which was moved medially on the anteroposterior radiographs at less than 6 months, 3 years, and final follow-up after operation.

70–140 degrees), whereas the mean abduction angle was 25 degrees (range, 15–40 degrees).

In all 28 hips, modified Merle d'Aubigne score was rated excellent in 11 hips, very good in 7 hips, good in 9 hips, and fair in 1 hip. In 26 hips without either recollapse or joint space narrowing, the score was rated excellent in 11 hips, very good in 7 hips, and good in 7 hips. One hip was rated fair because of poor motion with apparent limping. Two hips with joint space narrowing showed good results. Of 22 hips with nontraumatic necrosis, the score was excellent in 9 hips, very good in 7, good in 8, and fair in 1. Of six hips with traumatic necrosis, the score was excellent in two hips, very good in three hips, and good in one hip.

DISCUSSION

The importance of joint preservation of femoral head osteonecrosis in young patients (less than 50 years of age) is widely recognized among orthopedic surgeons. Joint-preserving procedures are usually effective in the case of small- or medium-sized lesions, and in early stage of the disease.[8–11] In the case of an extensive lesion, however, femoral head collapse usually occurs within a short period.[1] In cases of apparent collapse, conventional anterior rotational osteotomy reported by Sugioka and coworkers[12] is effective if the posterior viable area still remains. In patients with large collapsed necrotic lesions, however, various types of prosthetic replacement need to be performed, although the results of prosthetic replacement for young patients are controversial.[3–6,22] The authors have found that many young patients who have extensive lesions with advanced collapse are out of indication for an anterior rotational osteotomy. In cases with a viable area still available, the viable area can be moved to the loaded portion below the acetabular roof by the use of a posterior rotational osteotomy including the high-degree posterior rotational osteotomy as described by the present authors.[14,16,17]

As for the posterior rotational osteotomy, the blood supply of the affected femoral head is maintained because the posterior column artery branched off from the femoral medial circumflex artery is shifted medially and is not under tension. This has been confirmed by the authors' angiographic studies.[15] A high-degree posterior rotational osteotomy can be performed on cases with an extensive lesion. In the present study, the authors observed a high rate of spherical contour regained after operation on severely collapsed necrotic femoral heads as a remodeling process of the lesion. Subchondral fractures of the postoperative medial femoral heads disappeared on postoperative anteroposterior radiographs. The authors believe that the reason for the regaining of spherical contour was the containment and congruency of the joint caused by the superior to anterolateral adequate viable area of the femoral head. Containment and congruency between the femoral head and the acetabulum was improved not only in the neutral position, but also in flexion of daily activities with this posterior rotational osteotomy. The authors confirmed that as a result of posterior rotational osteotomy the anterior viable area was placed in the weight-bearing area below the acetabular roof in a flexed position seen on the 45 degrees flexion anteroposterior radiographs.[14,16,17] The previous reports of the results of posterior rotational osteotomy described by Atsumi and colleagues[14,16,17] showed good results if anterior viable extensive area was transferred to loaded portion below the acetabular roof. It is thought that one of the reasons for the good results was a respherical contour of the medial collapsed lesion as remodeling occurs.

SUMMARY

The authors believe that if adequate viable area can be placed under the loaded portion of the acetabulum and recollapse is prevented, the spherical contour of medial collapsed lesion can be regained as a result of remodeling. This might be one of the important factors in delaying the progression of degeneration after this posterior rotation osteotomy procedure, which can save the hips of young patients with extensive necrosis.

REFERENCES

1. Ohzono K, Saito M, Sugano N, et al. The fate of nontraumatic avascular necrosis of the femoral head: a radiologic classification to formulate prognosis. Clin Orthop Relat Res 1992;277:73–8.

2. Aubigne Merle d', Postel M, Mazabraud A, et al. Idiopathic necrosis of the femoral head in adults. J Bone Joint Surg Br 1965;47:612–33.

3. Adili A, Trousdale T. Femoral head resurfacing for the treatment of osteonecrosis in the young patient. Clin Orthop Relat Res 2003;417:93–101.

4. Chandler HP, Reineck FT, Wixson RL, et al. Total hip replacement in younger than thirty years old. J Bone Joint Surg Am 1981;63:1426–34.

5. Cornell NC, Salvati AE, Pelleicci PM. Long-term follow-up of total hip replacement in patients with osteonecrosis. Orthop Clin North Am 1985;16:757–69.

6. Garino JP, Steinberg ME. Total hip arthroplasty in patients with avascular necrosis of the femoral head. Clin Orthop Relat Res 1997;334:108–15.

7. Steinburg ME, Heyken GD, Steinburg DR. A quantitative system for staging avascular necrosis. J Bone Joint Surg Br 1995;77:34–41.

8. Fairbank AC, Bhatia D, Jinnah RH, et al. Long-term results of core decompression for ischemic necrosis of the femoral head. J Bone Joint Surg Br 1995;77:42–9.

9. Mont MA, Fairbank AC, Krackow KA, et al. Corrective osteotomy for osteonecrosis of the femoral head. J Bone Joint Surg Am 1996;78:1032–8.

10. Mont MA, Jones LC, Pacheco I, et al. Radiographic predictors of outcome of core decompression for hips with osteonecrosis stage III. Clin Orthop Relat Res 1998;354:159–68.

11. Urbaniak JR, Coogan PG, Gunneson EB, et al. Treatment of osteonecrosis of the femoral head with free vascularized fibular grafting: a long-term follow-up study of one hundred and three hips. J Bone Joint Surg Am 1995;77:681–94.

12. Sugioka Y, Hotokebuti T, Tsutsui H. Transtrochanteric anterior rotational osteotomy for idiopathic and steroid-induced necrosis of the femoral head: indications and long-term results. Clin Orthop Relat Res 1992;227:111–20.

13. Sugioka Y. Transtrochanteric rotational osteotomy of the femoral head. In: Riley Jr. LH, editor. The hip. Presented at the Proceedings of the eighth open scientific meeting of the hip society. St. Louis (MO), C.V. Mosby, 1980. p. 3–23.

14. Atsumi T, Kuroki Y. Modified Sugioka's osteotomy: more than 130° posterior rotation for osteonecrosis

15. Atsumi T, Yamano K. Superselective angiography in osteonecrosis of the femoral head. In: Urbaniak JR, Jones JP, editors. Osteonecrosis: etiology, diagnosis and treatment. American Academy of Orthopaedic Surgeons; 1997. p. 247–52.

16. Atsumi T, Muraki M, Yoshihara S, et al. Posterior rotational osteotomy for the treatment of femoral head osteonecrosis. Arch Orthop Trauma Surg 1999;119:388–93.

17. Atsumi T, Kajiwara T, Hiranuma Y, et al. Posterior rotational osteotomy for nontraumatic osteonecrosis with extensive collapsed lesions in young patients. J Bone Joint Surg Am 2006;88:42–7.

18. Sugano N, Atsumi T, Ohzono K, et al. The 2001 revised criteria for diagnosis, classification, and staging of idiopathic osteonecrosis of the femoral head. J Orthop Sci 2002;7:801–5.

19. Gardeniers JWM. ARCO committee on terminology and staging. ARCO News Letter 1993;5:79–82.

20. Atsumi T, Hosalkar H. Osteonecrosis of the hip. Tech Orthop 2008;23:54–64.

21. Moed BR, WillsonCarr SE, Watson JT. Results of operative treatment of fractures of the posterior wall of the acetabulum. J Bone Joint Surg Am 2002;84:752–8.

22. Piston RW, Engh CA. Osteonecrosis of the femoral head treated with total hip arthroplasty without cement. J Bone Joint Surg Am 1994;76:202–14.

Current Status of Hemi-Resurfacing Arthroplasty for Osteonecrosis of the Hip: A 27-Year Experience

Harlan C. Amstutz, MD*, Michel J. Le Duff, MA

KEYWORDS

- Hip • Hemiresurfacing • Osteonecrosis
- Long term • Survivorship • Outcome

Our experience with hemi-resurfacing arthroplasty for young patients with osteonecrosis of the femoral head began in the early 1980s, when we were disappointed with the durability of total hip arthroplasty (THA)[1–3] and surface arthroplasty with polyethylene.[4] Alternative treatment options, such as free vascularized fibula for collapsed femoral heads,[5] stemmed hemi-arthroplasty, which resulted in a substantial incidence of protrusio,[6] and our own experience and that of others with osteotomies,[7,8] also yielded less-than-satisfactory clinical results. Hemi-resurfacing offered a conservative prosthetic option because of its bone-preserving nature and the absence of wear debris–induced osteolysis (because no artificial bearing is inserted). Although some patients fail to obtain complete pain relief, hemi-resurfacing of the femoral head only was and still remains—an attractive alternative for young patients with stages II and III osteonecrosis and occasionally for young patients with early stage IV osteonecrosis (with minimal acetabular cartilage changes).

It was anticipated that the procedure would be "time buying" because the acetabular cartilage was damaged to a variable degree and would wear out in time. As such, the procedure was considered the first step of a lifetime treatment plan of young patients with anticipated conversion to full resurfacing or THA when improved bearing materials and design would be available. Fortunately, this evolution has occurred; new bearing technology and designs have provided better options with less wear, enhancing the durability of THA and full hip resurfacing. Because of these improvements, it is important to reassess the role and indications for hemi-resurfacing among the variety of prosthetic options available to the surgeon.

The purpose of the study discussed in this article was to review our long-term experience with this procedure, compare our clinical results to those of other centers, in particular regarding the difficulty of predicting pain relief, and determine the role of hemi-resurfacing in the future.

MATERIALS AND METHODS

Between February 1981 and December 2004, the senior author (HCA) treated 54 hips with a hemi-resurfacing device in a selected group of 46 patients with hip osteonecrosis. There were 12 women and

Funding for this study was provided by St Vincent Medical Center, Los Angeles, and Wright Medical Technologies Inc.

Joint Replacement Institute at St. Vincent Medical Center, Los Angeles, The S. Mark Taper Building, 2200 West Third Street, Suite 400, Los Angeles, CA 90057, USA

* Corresponding author. Medical Director, Joint Replacement Institute, The S. Mark Taper Building, 2200 West Third Street, Suite 400, Los Angeles, CA 90057, USA.

E-mail address: harlanamstutz@dochs.org (H.C. Amstutz).

Orthop Clin N Am 40 (2009) 275–282
doi:10.1016/j.ocl.2008.12.001

34 men. The mean age of patients was 34 years (range, 18–52), and their mean weight was 75 kg (range, 40–120). From the preoperative radiologic assessment we identified 4 hips with Ficat stage II osteonecrosis, 44 with Ficat stage III osteonecrosis, and 6 with early Ficat stage IV osteonecrosis. The risk factors for hip osteonecrosis included the use of corticosteroids (24 hips, 6 in patients with systemic lupus erythematosus), alcohol (11 hips), hip trauma (13 hips), idiopathic osteonecrosis (4 hips), and Gaucher's disease (2 hips). Sixteen patients were Charnley class A, 23 were Charnley class B, and 7 were Charnley class C. The mean time between the appearance of symptoms and the surgery was 11. 5 months (range, 2–39). The femoral head was photographed after preparation before cementing and in many instances the articular cartilage was photographed. The first 17 hips underwent operation with a transtrochanteric approach; the remaining 37 hips underwent operation with a posterior approach (since 1993). Three different component materials were used over time, with four different designs (**Fig. 1**). Eleven hips were resurfaced with a custom titanium alloy component (Zimmer, Warsaw, IN), 32 with a cobalt chromium molybdenum component (2 THARIES femoral shells, Zimmer, Warsaw, IN and 30 Conserve, Wright Medical Technology Inc., Arlington, TN), and 11 with a ceramic (Alumina) component (Kinamed Inc., Newbury Park, CA). In all cases, the femoral head was shaped as a chamfered cylinder. One component was press-fit (one of the alumina components), and the remaining cases were cemented.

The data collection consisted of a clinical evaluation using the UCLA hip score,[9,10] a four-item scale (pain, walking, function, and activity) graded from 1 to 10, in which 10 represents the best result (eg, no pain), and radiographs taken during the patient follow-up visits. Patients who were not able to come to our clinic received follow-up phone calls after mailing to our center radiographs performed locally. Four patients (6 hips) were lost to follow-up before 2 years and, at the time of our review, 6 patients had died of causes unrelated to the surgery, with an average follow-up time of 11 years (range, 3–13).

Indications for Hemi-Resurfacing

The indications included young patients who generally had osteonecrosis of Ficat II-III or early stage IV and radiographic preservation of some hip joint space. We included hips with large "whole head" lesions. The acetabular cartilage was assessed and the cartilage changes graded according to the classification presented by Beaulé and colleagues (**Table 1**).[11]

Surgical Technique

The surgical technique of the procedure was described previously,[12,13] but the principles of bone preparation and cementation are briefly

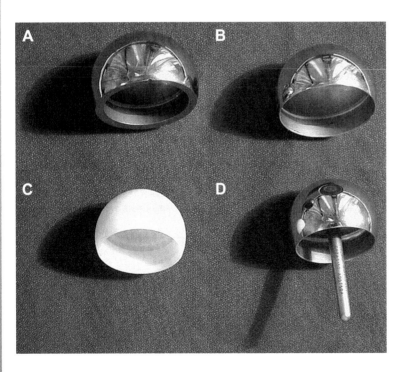

Fig. 1. The four different prosthetic designs used throughout our experience with hemi-resurfacing. (*A*) Titanium alloy custom component (Zimmer, Warsaw, IN). (*B*) THARIES CoCr femoral component (Zimmer, Warsaw, IN). (*C*) Custom Alumina component (Kinamed Inc., Newbury Park, CA). (*D*) Conserve CoCr component (Wright Medical Technology Inc., Arlington, TN).

Table 1
Acetabular cartilage grading based on its appearance and changes

Grade	Description	
I	Minimal changes, localized softening with some or no break in the surface. A blunt instrument pressed on the surface may sink into the cartilage. The cartilage may appear slightly discolored and soft	
II	Area of fissuring and irregular surface	
III	Definite fibrillation with fissuring extending down to subchondral bone	
	a	No osteophytes
	b	Noncalcified osteophytes
IV	Exposure and/or erosion of subchondral bone	

From Beaulé P, Schmalzried T, Campbell P, et al. Duration of symptoms and outcome of hemiresurfacing for hip osteonecrosis. Clin Orthop 2001;385:104–17; with permission.

emphasized here because they are critical for promoting intimate apposition of the cement with histologically viable bone. Although some changes in technique have occurred during the 23-year period, such as the approach, instrumentation, and thoroughness of cleaning and drying, the fundamental principles have not changed. All of the dead, yellowish, friable necrotic bone was removed with a curette and high-speed bur down to the more normal or dense white reactive bone, which was achieved by alternating burring, irrigation, and drying. This process led to substantial loss of the head in severe cases, but generally some portion of the cylindrically reamed bone remained, which was helpful for preserving leg length. Once this debridement was completed, the bone was penetrated with multiple 3-mm drill holes to increase the area for acrylic fixation. After the bone was optimally prepared, the acrylic was pressurized into the available cylindrically reamed cancellous bone and into the stem hole (for the Conserve components), and the component was fully seated.

Statistical Analysis

The Wilcoxon signed-rank test was used to compare preoperative to postoperative UCLA hip scores. Kaplan-Meier survival estimates[14] were used to determine the survivorship of the procedure, using the time to conversion to THA as the end point. The Cox proportional hazard ratio[15] was used to assess the influence of the following variables on the survivorship of the procedure: acetabular cartilage grade,[11] age at surgery, duration of symptoms before surgery, resurfacing material used, component size, patient weight, Ficat staging, and patient postoperative UCLA activity score. Spearmans' rank correlation coefficients were computed to study the effect of these variables on pain scores after surgery.

RESULTS

The mean follow-up time was 14 years (range 4–28). Preoperatively, the mean UCLA hip scores were 4.8 ± 1.8, 5.8 ± 1.8, 5.2 ± 1.6, and 4.2 ± 1.3 for pain, walking, function, and activity, respectively. At last follow-up, the mean UCLA hip scores were 8.0 ± 1.6, 8.9 ± 1.2, 7.9 ± 2.0, and 5.7 ± 1.4 for the hips that had not been revised. These scores were all significantly greater than the preoperative scores ($P < .0001$). These clinical scores are lower on average than those obtained in our cohort of patients treated with full metal-on-metal resurfacing for osteonecrosis (mean 9.4 ± 0.9, 9.4 ± 1.1, 9.3 ± 1.4, and 7.0 ± 1.7 for pain, walking, function, and activity, respectively).[16] The highest UCLA pain scores recorded for each patient averaged 8.6 ± 1.4. Two patients reported a highest pain score of 5, and three patients reported a score of 6, but 12 hips were rated at the maximum score of 10. We found a weak correlation between maximum pain score and the age of the patient at surgery (Spearman rho 0.328, $P = .024$). None of the other variables studied had any predictive value on the postoperative level of pain relief.

Range of Motion

The preoperative and postoperative range of motion measurements are summarized in **Table 2**. There was a minimal reduction in flexion, which was not significant, but improvements in abduction, adduction, and rotation were significant. All motion normalized postoperatively.

Radiographic Results

The last follow-up radiographs revealed no lesions that could have been interpreted as periprosthetic osteolysis. There has been no component

Table 2
Mean values of range of motion measured preoperatively and at the last follow-up

	Flexion	Flexion Contracture	Abduction (in Extension)	Adduction (in Extension)	Rotation Arc (in Extension)
Preoperatively	122.7 ± 12.5	6.4 ± 10.7	34.5 ± 14.9	22.2 ± 8.4	50.6 ± 23.1
Postoperatively	121.6 ± 12.6	3.0 ± 7.5	44.0 ± 8.4	28.8 ± 7.1	72.8 ± 17.9
p	0.770	0.251	0.005	0.013	0.004

loosening or radiographic evidence of neck narrowing. No cases of acetabular protrusion have been reported. Changes observed on serial radiographs included bone formation in the acetabular fossa (22 hips). We regarded this finding as a positive sign, which is associated with a longer survival of the procedure ($P = .0081$) (**Fig. 2**; see **Fig. 5**). After a variable period of time, however, the cartilage space narrows and may cause onset of pain, leading to a necessary revision.

Revisions

Twenty-three hips in 22 patients underwent revision surgery. One hip had a deep infection at 3 months that was treated at another facility with a two-stage THA. All the other revisions were secondary to wear of the host acetabular cartilage at an average of 8.2 years (range 0.7–23.2). Two hips were converted to metal-on-metal ConservePlus Resurfacing at 2.5 and 4 years by removing the alumina hemi-femoral component. Both are doing well 10.5 and 11 years after conversion, with UCLA scores of 10, 10, 8, and 7 and 10, 9, 10, and 7 for pain, walking, function, and activity, respectively. Two other hips were converted to a full hip resurfacing, keeping the femoral component in situ: one had a ConservePlus metal-on-metal bearing and the other had a metal-on-cross-linked polyethylene custom socket that was cemented into the acetabulum. The clinical results of these conversions are comparable to those of metal-on-metal resurfacing 3 and 8 years after revision surgery. The 19 remaining revisions were conversions to total hip replacements, 10 of which were performed at other facilities.

Complications

One patient suffered deep venous thrombosis of the contralateral leg 11 weeks after surgery, which resolved after treatment with heparin and Coumadin (the patient was initially treated postoperatively with Fragmin rather than our usual postoperative Coumadin regimen). No dislocations, femoral neck fractures, bleeding, heterotopic bone, nerve palsy, femoral component loosening, or other complications were reported in this series.

Survivorship

Using the time to revision surgery for any reason as endpoint, the Kaplan-Meier survival estimates were 79.6% (95% confidence interval 65.2%–88.5%) at 5 years, 63.3% (95% confidence interval 45.0%–77.0%) at 10 years, and 36.4% (95% confidence interval 17.3%–55.9%) at 15 years. The survivorship curve of the series is shown in **Fig. 3**. Additional time-dependant studies showed no difference in survivorship between component

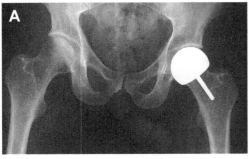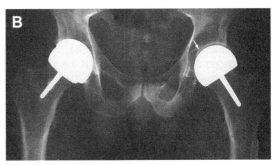

Fig. 2. (*A*) Anteroposterior radiograph of a 42-year-old man operated with the Conserve (Wright Medical Technology, Inc.) hemi-resurfacing component. (*B*) Four years after surgery, the component is well fixed and the acetabular cartilage preserved. The patient's UCLA pain score is 7. New bone formation is visible in the acetabular fossa (*arrow*). During this lapse of time, the patient underwent full metal-on-metal resurfacing on the contralateral side.

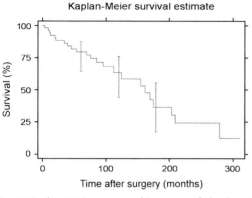

Fig. 3. Kaplan–Meier survivorship curve of the hemi-resurfacing prostheses implanted by the senior author (HCA). The time to revision for any reason was used as end point. Ninety-five percent confidence intervals are indicated at 5, 10, and 15 years.

materials (P = .944). We found no association between time to revision and Ficat staging (P = .710), the duration of symptoms before surgery (P = .321), patient weight (P = .234), patient activity (P = .291), or femoral component size (P = .826). An acetabular cartilage grade of IIIa or more and a lower age of the patient at surgery were related to a shorter time to revision (**Table 3**).

DISCUSSION

The clinical results and rates of survivorship in this group of hemi-resurfacing procedures are consistent with those reported by other authors.[17,18] We anticipated improved results with the alumina or cobalt chrome shells over titanium alloy because of surface scratches observed during the revision of those relatively soft components. Because of the hydrophilic nature of the smooth alumina surface, we hoped that the wear of the cartilage would diminish, but survivorship results have been comparable regardless of the materials used. We suspect that the dominant negative physical property of the femoral component responsible for cartilage wear is its hardness

compared with that of the cartilage, especially if this cartilage is not normal.

Because of its brittle nature, the alumina component had one advantage over components made of metal because the component could be split and removed with minimal bone loss and a full metal-on-metal resurfacing subsequently could be performed when revision was needed. It is not possible to remove metal femoral components without substantial bone loss of an already compromised femoral head, and conversion requires a THA. Currently, the CoCr ConservePlus femoral component used for hemi-resurfacing is prepared with tolerances designed for metal-on-metal bearings so that a conversion can be performed by inserting a socket (**Fig. 4**). The acetabulum must have a wall thickness sufficient to accommodate the socket, however, and this option is more likely to be appropriate for male patients than female patients, who generally present with thinner acetabular wall thickness. Although hemi-resurfacing clinical scores from the current study are not as good as those for full resurfacing,[19,20] they are comparable or better than those from our experience with osteotomy[7] or the reported results from grafting procedures.[21]

Osteonecrosis patients (particularly patients who have had a short duration of symptoms, as generally has been the case with patients undergoing hemi-resurfacing) typically present with a relatively minimal restriction of range of motion preoperatively, except for a consistent loss of internal rotation and some Abduction/adduction. The postoperative range of motion normalizes and is not different than that for patients who undergo full resurfacing.[16] Most patients are satisfied with the outcome. Patients frequently report that the pain relief is not a 9 or 10 on the pain scale initially, but it generally improves with time until the moment when the cartilage wears out. Our longest survivor has undergone 27 years of follow-up after hemi-resurfacing for Ficat III and is an example of this pattern (**Fig. 5**). Four patients required a revision within the first 14 months after surgery, however, which in each instance resulted from

Table 3
Effect of the variables related to a shorter prosthetic survival

	Hazard Ratio	p	95% Confidence Interval
Acetabular cartilage grading	2.701011	0.055	[0.9790394–7.45165]
Age at surgery	0.5513417	0.017	[0.3382122–0.898778]

The Cox proportional hazard ratio was calculated with mutual adjustment (multivariate model). The acetabular cartilage grading was studied as low grades (I and II) versus high grades (IIIa, IIIb, and IV). Age at surgery was studied by groups of 10 years.

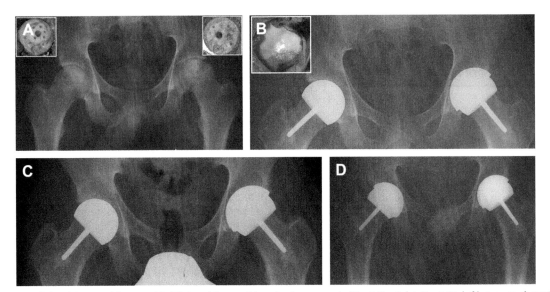

Fig. 4. (*A*) A 24-year-old man with bilateral femoral head osteonecrosis (Ficat III, *right*; Ficat IV, *left*). Inserts show intraoperative photographs taken at the end of the preparation phase of the femoral head. (*B*) The patient is shown 1 month after one-stage bilateral hip arthroplasty. A total hip resurfacing with a 50 mm femoral head and 56 mm socket was performed on the left hip and a hemi-resurfacing of 50 mm (slightly undersized) was performed on the right. The insert shows an intraoperative photograph of the acetabular cartilage on the right hip, graded IIIa. Note preosteophytes inferiorly. Both stems were cemented. (*C*) Eleven months postoperatively, the acetabular cartilage of the right hip is clearly obliterated. The patient's UCLA scores are 5, 7, 7, 6 for pain, walking, function, and activity, respectively. In retrospect, the acetabular cartilage of the right hip was probably too damaged to anticipate buying a significant amount of time before conversion, and reoperation was needed after only a year. (*D*) The patient is shown 9 months after conversion of the right hip to full resurfacing and 20 months postoperatively (on the left). He has returned to a normal quality of life with UCLA hip scores of 10, 10, 8, and 7 for pain, walking, function, and activity, respectively, for both hips. (*From* Amstutz HC. Hip resurfacing, principles, indications, technique, and results. Philadelphia: Saunders–Elsevier; 2008. p. 170.)

rapid cartilage wear that can be attributed to extending the indications and accepting more cartilage damage (grade III and IV) in young patients. Two of our patients who were less satisfied than most others (reporting incomplete pain relief of 6 and 8 on the UCLA scale) had bilateral disease in which one side received a hemi-resurfacing device and the contralateral side received a full resurfacing (which did provide complete pain relief). When the patients were reminded of the "time buying" objectives of the hemi-resurfacing procedure, they seemed to understand the reason for not implanting full bearing couples in both hips at a young age and are satisfied 7 and 9 years after surgery. Our young patients are often more demanding than in the past and may be less tolerant of pain and the relative difficulty or inadvisability of participating in physical activities in a manner similar to that of their peers. For hemi-resurfacing to be successful, patients must buy into the concept of "time buying."

Hemi-resurfacing remains our preference for young patients (< 30 years of age) who have selected cases with Ficat II and III and good acetabular cartilage. The justification for hemi-resurfacing at that time is the avoidance of a procedure with potentially adverse consequences, such as the possible effects of metal ions and wear in metal-on-metal bearings, the squeaking and component fractures associated with ceramic bearings, and the unknown potential for osteolysis or long-term durability of cross-linked polyethylene. The latter two bearing materials are used with THA, whereas currently, metal-on-metal bearings are the only available solution for hip resurfacing. The use of cross-linked polyethylene bearings and all ceramic devices poses some restrictions on femoral head size, and their stability is inferior to that of the larger balls in metal-on-metal devices. We do not recommend hemi-resurfacing for older patients, however, because of the current success of full metal-on-metal resurfacing for osteonecrosis.[22,23]

From our experience, hemi-resurfacing is not indicated for patients who must do work that involves standing and walking on hard cement floors, patients involved in workman's compensation cases, or patients who do not understand the limited objectives of pain relief and return to normal function. Our recent hemi-resurfacing procedures have been performed exclusively

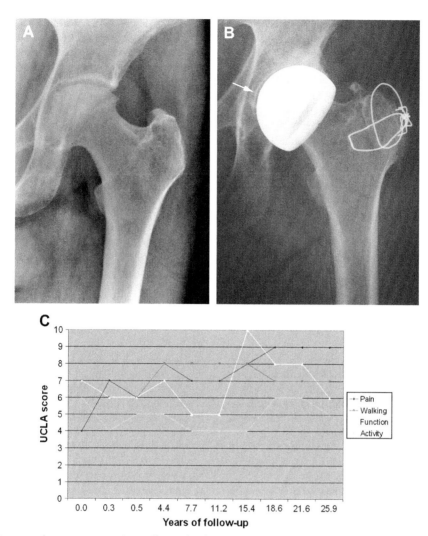

Fig. 5. (*A*) Preoperative anteroposterior radiograph of a 35-year-old woman with systemic lupus erythematosis/steroid-induced osteonecrosis Ficat stage III of the left hip. (*B*) Same patient 26 years after hemi-resurfacing. There is new bone formation in the acetabular fossa. The acetabular cartilage has narrowed, especially superiorly, and there is increased density of the bone in the acetabulum superior to the joint, but the patient still has minimal pain. (*C*) Plot of the patient's UCLA hip scores over time. (*From* Amstutz HC. Hip resurfacing, principles, indications, technique, and results. Philadelphia: Saunders–Elsevier; 2008. p. 167)

with the ConservePlus Femoral components, which have the ability to convert to full resurfacing if necessary. It is not known if this is an option with other resurfacing systems. From the results of this study showing the difficulty to predict the level of pain relief after hemi-resurfacing and the experience of other researchers,[17] it seems unrealistic to expect postoperative clinical scores as high as those obtained with full resurfacing in every case. Patients should be informed fully and accept the "time-buying" objectives of the procedure before undergoing surgery. For a large proportion of our patients, this strategy has been successful, and with several patients a surprisingly long durability has been achieved (**Fig. 5**).

REFERENCES

1. Cornell CN, Salvati EA, Pellicci PM, et al. Long-term follow-up of total hip replacement in patients with osteonecrosis. Orthop Clin North Am 1985;16:757–69.
2. Saito S, Saito M, Tetsuhiko N, et al. Long-term results of total hip arthroplasty for osteonecrosis of the femoral head. Clin Orthop Relat Res 1989;244:198–207.
3. Piston RW, Engh CA, De Carvalho PI, et al. Osteonecrosis of the femoral head treated with total hip arthroplasty without cement. J Bone Joint Surg Am 1994;76A(2):202–14.
4. Dutton R, Amstutz H, Thomas B, et-al. THARIES surface replacement for osteonecrosis of the femoral head. J Bone Joint Surg Am 1982;64(A)3:1225–37.

5. Marciniak D, Furey C, Shaffer J, et al. Osteonecrosis of the femoral head: a study of 101 hips treated with vascularized fibular grafting. J Bone Joint Surg Am 2005;87(4):742–7.

6. Ito H, Matsuno T, Kaneda K, et al. Bipolar hemiarthroplasty for osteonecrosis of the femoral head: a 7- to 18-year followup. Clin Orthop 2000;374: 201–11 [In Process Citation].

7. Tooke SM, Amstutz HC, Hedley AK, et al. Results of transtrochanteric rotational osteotomy for femoral head osteonecrosis. Clin Orthop 1987;224:150–7.

8. Dean MT, Cabanela ME. Transtrochanteric anterior rotational osteotomy for avascular necrosis of the femoral head: long-term results. J Bone Joint Surg Br 1993;75:597–601 A(B).

9. Amstutz H, Thomas B, Jinnah R, et al. Treatment of primary osteoarthritis of the hip: a comparison of total joint and surface replacement arthroplasty. J Bone Joint Surg 1984;66A(2):228–41.

10. Naal F, Impellizzeri F, Leunig M, et al. Which is the best activity rating scale for patients undergoing total joint arthroplasty? Clin Orthop Relat Res 2009; 467(4):958–65.

11. Beaulé P, Schmalzried T, Campbell P, et al. Duration of symptoms and outcome of hemiresurfacing for hip osteonecrosis. Clin Orthop 2001;385:104–17.

12. Beaulé P, Amstutz H. Hemiresurfacing arthroplasty for osteonecrosis of the hip. Operative Techniques in Orthopaedics 2000;10(2):123–32.

13. Tooke SM, Amstutz HC, Delaunay C, et al. Hemiresurfacing for femoral head osteonecrosis. J Arthroplasty 1987;2–2:125–33.

14. Kaplan E, Meier P. Nonparametric estimation from incomplete observations. J Am Stat Assoc 1958; 53:457–81.

15. Cox D. Regression models and life tables. Journal of the Royal Statistical Society 1972;34:187–220.

16. Amstutz H, Le Duff M, Boitano P, et al. Osteonecrosis of the hip. In: Amstutz HC, editor. Hip resurfacing: principles, indications, technique and results Philadelphia: Elsevier; 2008. p. 161–80.

17. Cuckler J, Moore K, Estrada L, et al. Outcome of hemiresurfacing in osteonecrosis of the femoral head. Clin Orthop Relat Res 2004;429 146–50.

18. Grecula M, Thomas J, Kreuzer S, et al. Impact of implant design on femoral head hemiresurfacing arthroplasty. Clin Orthop Relat Res 2004;418 41–7.

19. Beaulé P, Amstutz H, Le Duff M, et al. Surface arthroplasty for osteonecrosis of the hip: Hemiresurfacing versus metal-on-metal hybrid resurfacing. J Arthroplasty 2004;19(12):54–8.

20. Amstutz H, Le Duff M. Eleven years of experience with metal-on-metal hybrid hip resurfacing: a review of 1000 conserve plus. J Arthroplasty 2008 23(6 Suppl. 1):36–43.

21. Scully SP, Aaron RK, Urbaniak JR, et al. Survival analysis of hips treated with core decompression or vascularized fibular grafting because of avascular necrosis. J Bone Joint Surg Am 1998 80A(9):1270–5.

22. Mont M, Seyler T, Marker D, et al. Use of metal-on-metal total hip resurfacing for the treatment of osteonecrosis of the femoral head. J Bone Joint Surg Am 2006;88(suppl 3):90–7.

23. Revell M, McBryde C, Bhatnagar S, et al. Metal-on-metal hip resurfacing in osteonecrosis of the femoral head. J Bone Joint Surg Am 2006;88(suppl 3) 98–103.

Outcome of Uncemented Primary Femoral Stems for Treatment of Femoral Head Osteonecrosis

Marc W. Hungerford, MD, David S. Hungerford, MD,
Lynne C. Jones, PhD*

KEYWORDS
- Hip arthroplasty • Treatment • Femoral head necrosis
- Hip prosthesis • Treatment outcome

Total hip replacement (THR) has been for several decades a safe and reliable treatment for end-stage osteoarthritis of the hip in older patients. As the indications have broadened to other disease states and to younger patient populations, the results of this procedure have not been as reliable. Osteonecrosis of the femoral head (ONFH) poses particular challenges to the joint replacement surgeon because many patients are relatively young, have normal activity levels, and have normal life expectancies. Also, many patients who are less active have comorbid conditions, such as systemic lupus erythematosus, that require chronic corticosteroid use, which can affect bone quality.

For these reasons, past reports on the outcomes of THR in this patient population have shown unsatisfactory results.[1–3] More recent reports using updated implant designs and modern cementation techniques have shown more encouraging outcomes (**Table 1**). In fact, osteonecrosis may not be an independe nt risk factor for survivorship in THR.[4,5]

Each member of the Porous Coated Anatomic (PCA) family of stems (Stryker Orthopaedics, Mahwah, New Jersey; formerly Howmedica) has a proximally coated, chrome-cobalt, anatomically shaped, press-fit design for use without cement. Clinically reported outcomes for this stem family have been good.[6–11] This study documents the outcomes for these stems in patients with osteonecrosis and examines any difference in outcome with successive generations of stem design.

MATERIALS AND METHODS
Demographics

During the period from 1983 to 1995, 158 cases of ONFH in 141 patients were treated with total hip arthroplasty at our institution using a stem from the PCA family of femoral stems. The PCA stem was first introduced in 1983 and through the period of study went through three iterations of development: PCA E-series, Meridian, and Citation. In this study group, there were 74 men and 67 women who had a mean age at index surgery of 46 years (range, 17–83 years). Their mean duration at follow-up was 103 months (range, 20–235 months). This study received Institutional Review Board approval.

The PCA group, the first and largest group in this series, involved 77 hips and 66 patients, including 34 men and 32 women. Their mean age at index surgery was 47 years (range, 19–83 years). Their mean follow-up interval was 124 months (range, 20–235 months). At the time of final follow-up, 18 of these patients had died; none of the deaths were related to surgery. Each of the patients who died by the time of final follow-up had a well-functioning prosthesis at the time of death.

Johns Hopkins Orthopaedics at Good Samaritan Hospital, Suite G-1 GSH Smyth Building, 5601 Loch Raven Boulevard, Baltimore, MD 21239, USA
* Corresponding author.
E-mail address: ljones3@jhmi.edu (L.C. Jones).

Orthop Clin N Am 40 (2009) 283–289
doi:10.1016/j.ocl.2008.10.006

Table 1
Series of THR in osteonecrosis patients (survivorship of femur; based on revision for aseptic loosening)

Investigators	Number of Hip Implants	Mean Follow-up	Survivorship (Aseptic Loosening)	Comment
Cornell and colleagues, 1985[16]	28 cemented	7.6 y	96.4%	
Devlin and colleagues, 1988[20]	36 cemented	7.2 yrs	86.1%	Renal transplant patients
Radford and colleagues, 1989[21]	31 cemented	6 yrs	93.5%	Renal transplant patients
Saito and colleagues, 1989[22]	29 cemented	7.2 y	79.3%	
Elke and Morscher, 1990[23]	52 cemented; 21 uncemented	4.9 y	96.2% (cemented); 85.7% (uncemented)	
Huo and colleagues, 1992[24]	26 cemented; 3 uncemented	4.3 y	96.2% (cemented); 100% (uncemented)	Systemic lupus erythematosus patients
Katz and colleagues, 1992[25]	20 cemented; 14 uncemented	4.7 y (cemented); 2.6 y (uncemented)	100% (cemented); 100% (uncemented)	
Lins and colleagues, 1993[26]	37 uncemented	4–6 y	100%	
Brinker and colleagues, 1994[27]	81 uncemented	5.7 y	92.6%	
Phillips and colleagues, 1994[28]	20 uncemented	5.2 y	100%	
Stulberg and colleagues, 1997[29]	87 uncemented	7.3 y	95.4%	
Garino and Steinberg, 1997[18]	123 cemented	4.6 y	98.4%	
Fye and colleagues, 1998[30]	66 uncemented	7 y	98.5%	
Hartley and colleagues, 2000[31]	48 uncemented	10.3 y	100%	
Xenakis and colleagues, 2001[32]	36 uncemented	11.2 y	100%	
Fyda and colleagues, 2002[33]	48 cemented	10 y minimum	90.9%	
Kim and colleagues, 2003[19]	50 cemented; 98 uncemented	9.3 y	100% cemented; 98% uncemented	
Mont and colleagues, 2006[34]	52 uncemented	3.1 y	98.1%	

E-series implants were placed in 47 hips of 43 patients. In this group were 25 men and 18 women. Their mean age at implantation was 45 years (range, 20–65 years). The mean time of follow-up was 105 months (range, 24–204 months). Six patients have died of unrelated causes. Each of those 6 had well-functioning implants at the time of death.

In the Meridian group, there were 18 hips in 17 patients, of which 9 were men and 8 were women. Their mean age at implantation was 49 years (range, 28–75 years). The mean time of follow-up was 69 months (range, 24–131 months). At the time of follow-up, 1 patient had died of causes unrelated to the hip; at their most recent follow-up visit (10 years), the prosthesis was well fixed and well functioning.

Among the 15 patients who received the Citation stem procedures performed most recently, there were 16 hips among 6 men and 9 women. Their mean age was 43 years (range, 17–59 years). The mean follow-up was 42 months (range, 24–82 months). There were no deaths in this group at the time of final follow-up.

Table 2 summarizes the demographics for each of the stem groups included in this study.

Stems

The design of all femoral stems in this series was based on that of the PCA or porous-coated anatomic hip stem (**Fig. 1**). This is a short, anatomically bowed, proximally flared and coated chrome-cobalt stem. The bow was designed to conform to the posterior bow of the femur. The proximal third is coated with three layers of sintered beads. This was a broach-only system with implantation and preparation of the proximal femur done with matching broaches. The stem was supplied in six sizes, and 32-mm heads were used. In this study, the PCA stem was used from 1983 to 1995. The PCA and all other stems in this family are collarless and made of Vitallium, a chrome-cobalt alloy. They have good metaphyseal fit and fill and each has been available with a modular head.

The E-series prosthesis was the first evolution of the PCA prosthesis (see **Fig. 1**). It is slightly modified in shape with an increased proximal flare, both laterally and posteriorly, to achieve better initial press-fit stability. Additionally, the posterior bow is slightly reshaped to reduce impingement of the tip on the anterior cortex of the femur. The stem is also slightly longer. Furthermore, it was available in nine sizes, rather than six for the PCA. The E-series and all subsequent series were used with 26-mm rather than 32-mm heads. The E-series was in use from 1990 to 1995.

The Meridian prostheses were a further evolution of the PCA family (see **Fig. 1**) and were implanted by our group from July 1995 until October 1996. This is, in fact, a straight stem rather than an anatomically bowed stem, but preserves the anatomic fit and fill characteristics of the proximal metaphysis pioneered by the PCA stem. It is also made of chrome-cobalt with its proximal third porous coated. Unlike earlier stems in this family, the distal two thirds of this stem are polished to reduce stress-shielding thought to be caused by on-growth of cortical bone onto the distal stem. It also has features designed to reduce the stiffness of the tip of the stem. Smaller stems are fluted and larger stems have a "clothes pin" slot in the coronal plane at the tip of the stem to reduce stiffness.

The Citation prosthesis, the most recent version of this family (1997–present), is an anatomically curved stem, again to match the posterior bow and retain the advanced features of the Meridian stem, including the distal stem-polishing and the stiffness-reduction features of the Meridian (see **Fig. 1**). The stem is also porous coated at its proximal end. It is used with 26-mm modular heads.

Both the Meridian and Citation stems are still available.

Table 2
Patient demographics

	PCA	E-series	Meridian	Citation
Number of cases (number of patients)	77 (66)	47 (43)	18 (17)	16 (15)
Men/women	34/32	25/18	9/8	6/9
Age	47 y (range, 19–83 y)	45 y (range, 20–65 y)	49 y (range, 28–75 y)	43 y (range, 17–59 y)
Mean follow-up	123.7 mo (range, 20–235 mo)	104.5 mo (range, 24–204 mo)	69.2 mo (range, 24–131 mo)	41.9 mo (range, 24–82 mo)

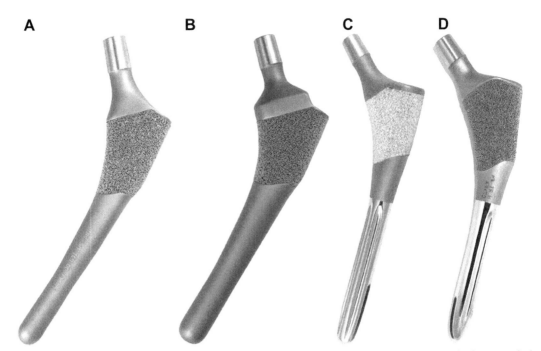

Fig. 1. Uncemented femoral stems evaluated in this study. (*A*) PCA: proximally porous coated; chrome-cobalt, anatomic posterior bow. (*B*) PCA E-series: slightly longer; increased posterior and lateral flare; more sizes. (*C*) Meridian: no posterior bow; distally polished; stiffness-reduction features at tip. (*D*) Citation: posterior bow; distally polished; stiffness-reduction features at tip.

Surgical Procedure and Follow-up Care

A modified Harding direct lateral approach in the decubitus position was used for all patients.[9] Postoperatively, all patients used protected 50% weight-bearing for the first 6 weeks. Each patient used bilateral support and followed hip dislocation precautions during this period. At 6 weeks, abductor strengthening was initiated and patients were permitted to bear weight as tolerated. Postoperatively, the patients were followed at 6 weeks, 3 months, 6 months, and yearly thereafter. Postoperative follow-up data collection consisted of a medical history, detailed physical examination, anteroposterior and lateral radiographs of the operated hip, and an anteroposterior radiograph of the pelvis. Harris hip scores and SF-36 quality-of-life scores were collected at the time of follow-up as was any information on reoperations, including revisions, and any complications during or after surgery.

Data Collection and Analysis

All data were recorded into an Institutional Review Board–approved Microsoft Access database. Statistical analysis was accomplished using the PEPI statistical software program (USD, Inc.,

Stone Mountain, Georgia). Chi-square analysis was performed in the analysis of differences in frequencies. Kaplan-Meier survival analysis was performed defining revision THR as "failure." A *P* value of .05 or less was accepted as statistically significant.

RESULTS

At the time of final follow-up, the average Harris hip score of the 144 unrevised cases improved from a mean of 45 ($\pm$17) points preoperatively to a mean of 84 ($\pm$15) points postoperatively. There were 14 revisions (8.9%) with 12 cases revised for femoral loosening or significant osteolysis, 1 case revised for deep infection, and 1 case revised for chronic dislocation. With respect to the revision rates for individual stems in the stem family, 9 of 77 PCA (12%) were revised with the mean time to revision of 73 months (range, 25–132 months). Two of 46 E-series implants (4.3%) were revised. The mean time to revision was 85 months (2 cases in one patient; 68 and 101 months respectively). For the Meridian stem, 2 of 18 were revised (11.1%) with the mean time to revision of 103 months (98 and 107 months, respectively). One of the 16 Citation stems was revised (6.3%) with the time to revision of 30 months.

In the PCA group, the mean Harris hip score for the unrevised patients at the time of final follow-up was 83 (±15) points. Of the nine revisions in this group, eight were revised for aseptic loosening and one patient was revised for a deep infection. The deep infection developed at 6 years' postprocedure.

With PCA E-series stems, the mean Harris hip score for the unrevised patients was 87 (±13) points. In this group, there were two revisions, both for aseptic loosening (4.3%). The mean Harris hip score for the unrevised patients with Meridian stems was 88 (±13) points at the time of final follow-up. There were two revisions in this group (11.1%): one for chronic dislocation and one for aseptic loosening of the femoral stem. The mean Harris hip score in the unrevised patients with Citation stems was 78 (±23) points. There were four poor results in this group. One patient had unexplained thigh pain, which had not resolved at 1-year postprocedure. One patient had moderate pain on the Harris hip score and some limitation in the range of motion of the operated hip. One patient had moderate pain in the contralateral hip, resulting in a severe limp. That patient required a crutch for ambulation. This was due to pain in the contralateral hip. Finally, one patient had severe pain due to low back pain and pain on the contralateral side. There was one revision in this group (6.3%) for aseptic loosening of the femoral stem.

Fig. 2 shows the revision rates for all four stems in this series. There was no significant difference in the revision rates for each stem. **Fig. 3** shows the Kaplan-Meier survivorship curves for all the stems in the stem family, while **Fig. 3** shows the stratified results. The survivorship result was 95.6% (95%

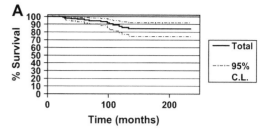

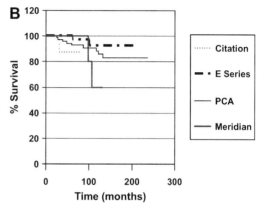

Fig. 3. Kaplan-Meier survivorship curves for (A) the pooled results for all stems included in this study and (B) the results stratified according to stem type. CL, confidence limits.

CI, 91.5–98.1%) at 5 years and 87.6% (95% CI 78.9–93.8%) at 10 years. No 10-year data was available at this time for the Citation prosthesis. Statistical analysis did not reveal any statistically significant differences in survivorship among the stems in the stem family.

DISCUSSION

End-stage ONFH has posed a difficult management challenge for the arthroplasty surgeon. Patients are typically young and otherwise healthy. Data available at the beginning of this study (1983) indicated that cemented THR had an unacceptably high rate of failure in young patients.[3,12,13] Radiographic analysis showed high rates of wear and severe osteolysis. At that time, osteolysis was attributed to the failure of the cement.[14] Early experience with the uncemented PCA, which we have previously published,[7] indicated good results for a mixed patient population. Given this history, the senior author hypothesized that biologic fixation gave the young osteonecrosis patient the most favorable outlook for a durable, functional result.

Outcomes for THR in patients with ONFH were decidedly less than optimal and compared poorly to outcomes in patients with osteoarthritis.[2,3] In

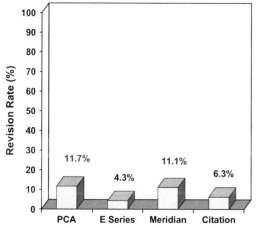

Fig. 2. Revision rates for the uncemented primary stems used in this study.

fact, 25 of 27 studies reviewed by Mont and Hungerford[1] in 1995 showed inferior results for patients with ONFH compared with those for matched groups with osteoarthritis. Reasons postulated for these inferior outcomes included the young age and high activity of the patients, the comorbid conditions in the osteonecrosis population (including systemic lupus erythematosus and rheumatoid arthritis), the continued use of corticosteroids in the osteonecrosis group, and the recognition that the bone abnormalities and necrosis that is seen in ONFH can extend to the metaphyseal region of the femur and therefore can affect stem fixation.[5,15–17]

Members of the PCA family of stems share certain common features. They are all made of chrome-cobalt, proximally porous coated with sintered beads for bony ingrowth, and designed to maximize fit and fill of the proximal femur. All are designed to be implanted without milling or reaming. With the exception of the Meridian femoral stem, all of these stems are curved in the coronal plane to conform to the proximal bow of the femur. The clinical outcomes reported for these stems by various investigators have been excellent. Kawamura and colleagues[8] reported 94.9% survivorship of the original PCA stem at 14-year follow-up. Bojescul and colleagues[6] reported 92% survivorship at 15-year average follow-up using the PCA stem. In younger patients, this stem family has enjoyed above-average performance. Mont and colleagues[9] reported 90% survivorship at 4.5-year average follow-up in patients under the age of 40. The next version, the PCA E-series, also proved clinically successful. Mont and colleagues[10] reported 98% survivorship at 5-year follow-up and Tankersley and colleagues[11] reported 95% survivorship over a similar follow-up period.

Although early reported outcomes for THR in patients with ONFH were poor, more recent studies using both cemented and cementless designs have reported results equivalent to those in age- and activity-matched patients with osteoarthritis. Garino and Steinberg[18] reported a 1.6% revision rate at 4.6-year average follow-up using the cemented Harris Design Two (HD-2) stem. Schneider and Knahr[4] reported no failures in 35 patients at 10-year follow-up using the Zweymueller prosthesis. Kim and colleagues[19] directly compared cementless to cemented stems in patients with ONFH. The investigators reported no revisions for aseptic loosening in either group at 9.5-year average follow-up.

Our results using the PCA family of stems in patients with ONFH compares favorably to the results seen with this design in patients with osteoarthritis, and with the use of other stem designs in patients with ONFH. We did note an improvement in outcome between the results from the original PCA design and the subsequent, improved designs retaining the anatomic design. The improvement could be attributed to design modifications yielding better rotational stability, to better fit and fill, or simply to increased experience with this style of stem and better surgical technique.

SUMMARY

Cementless THR has been advocated for the younger, more active patient, such as those with ONFH. The PCA series of stems led to excellent long-term clinical results when used in patients who require THR because of ONFH.

ACKNOWLEDGMENTS

The authors wish to thank Patricia Pietryak and Amy Jones for their technical assistance with the data collection for this manuscript.

REFERENCES

1. Mont MA, Hungerford DS. Non-traumatic avascular necrosis of the femoral head. J Bone Joint Surg 1995;77:459–74.
2. Salvati EA, Cornell CN. Long-term follow-up of total hip replacement in patients with avascular necrosis. Instr Course Lect 1988;37:67–73.
3. Stauffer RN. Ten-year follow-up study of total hip replacement. J Bone Joint Surg 1982;64:983–90.
4. Schneider W, Knahr K. Total hip replacement in younger patients: survival rate after avascular necrosis of the femoral head. Acta Orthop Scand 2004;75: 142–6.
5. Seyler TM, Cui Q, Mihalko WM, et al. Advances in hip arthroplasty in the treatment of osteonecrosis. Instr Course Lect 2007;56:221–33.
6. Bojescul JA, Xenos JS, Callaghan JJ, et al. Results of porous-coated anatomic total hip arthroplasty without cement at fifteen years: a concise follow-up of a previous report. J Bone Joint Surg 2003;85-A: 1079–83.
7. Hedley AK, Gruen TA, Borden LS, et al. Two-year follow-up of the PCA noncemented total hip replacement. Hip 1987;225–50.
8. Kawamura H, Dunbar MJ, Murray P, et al. The porous coated anatomic total hip replacement. A ten to fourteen-year follow-up study of a cementless total hip arthroplasty. J Bone Joint Surg 2001;83-A: 1333–8.
9. Mont MA, Maar DC, Krackow KA, et al. Total hip replacement without cement for non-inflammatory osteoarthrosis in patients who are less than forty-five years old. J Bone Joint Surg 1993;75:740–51.

10. Mont MA, Yoon TR, Krackow KA, et al. Clinical experience with a proximally porous-coated second-generation cementless total hip prosthesis: minimum 5-year follow-up. J Arthroplasty 1999;14:930–9.

11. Tankersley WS, Mont MA, Hungerford DS. A second-generation cementless hip prosthesis: improved results over the first-generation prosthesis. Am J Orthop 1997;26:839–44.

12. Collis DK. Cemented total hip replacement in patients who are less than fifty years old. J Bone Joint Surg 1984;66:353–9.

13. Dorr LD, Takei GK, Conaty JP. Total hip arthroplasties in patients less than forty-five years old. J Bone Joint Surg 1983;65:474–9.

14. Jones LC, Hungerford DS. Cement disease. Clin Orthop Relat Res 1987;225:192–206.

15. Calder JD, Pearse MF, Revell PA. The extent of osteocyte death in the proximal femur of patients with osteonecrosis of the femoral head. J Bone Joint Surg Br 2001;83:419–22.

16. Cornell CN, Salvati EA, Pellicci PM. Long-term follow-up of total hip replacement in patients with osteonecrosis. Orthop Clin North Am 1985;16:757–69.

17. Sarmiento A, Ebramzadeh E, Gogan WJ, et al. Total hip arthroplasty with cement. A long-term radiographic analysis in patients who are older than fifty and younger than fifty years. J Bone Joint Surg 1990;72:1470–6.

18. Garino JP, Steinberg ME. Total hip arthroplasty in patients with avascular necrosis of the femoral head: a 2- to 10-year follow-up. Clin Orthop Relat Res 1997;334:108–15.

19. Kim YH, Oh SH, Kim JS, et al. Contemporary total hip arthroplasty with and without cement in patients with osteonecrosis of the femoral head. J Bone Joint Surg 2003;85-A:675–81.

20. Devlin VJ, Einhorn TA, Gordon SL, et al. Total hip arthroplasty after renal transplantation. Long-term follow-up study and assessment of metabolic bone status. J Arthroplasty 1988;3:205–13.

21. Radford PJ, Doran A, Greatorex RA, et al. Total hip replacement in the renal transplant recipient. J Bone Joint Surg Br 1989;71:456–9.

22. Saito S, Saito M, Nishina T, et al. Long-term results of total hip arthroplasty for osteonecrosis of the femoral head. A comparison with osteoarthritis. Clin Orthop Relat Res 1989;244:198–207.

23. Elke R, Morscher E. [Total prosthesis arthroplasty in femur head necrosis]. Orthopade 1990;19:236–41.

24. Huo MH, Salvati EA, Browne MG, et al. Primary total hip arthroplasty in systemic lupus erythematosus. J Arthroplasty 1992;7:51–6.

25. Katz RL, Bourne RB, Rorabeck CH, et al. Total hip arthroplasty in patients with avascular necrosis of the hip. Follow-up observations on cementless and cemented operations. Clin Orthop Relat Res 1992;281:145–51.

26. Lins RE, Barnes BC, Callaghan JJ, et al. Evaluation of uncemented total hip arthroplasty in patients with avascular necrosis of the femoral head. Clin Orthop Relat Res 1993;297:168–73.

27. Brinker MR, Rosenberg AG, Kull L, et al. Primary total hip arthroplasty using noncemented porous-coated femoral components in patients with osteonecrosis of the femoral head. J Arthroplasty 1994;9:457–68.

28. Phillips FM, Pottenger LA, Finn HA, et al. Cementless total hip arthroplasty in patients with steroid-induced avascular necrosis of the hip. A 62-month follow-up study. Clin Orthop Relat Res 1994;303:147–54.

29. Stulberg BN, Singer R, Goldner J, et al. Uncemented total hip arthroplasty in osteonecrosis: a 2- to 10-year evaluation. Clin Orthop Relat Res 1997;334:116–23.

30. Fye MA, Huo MH, Zatorski LE, et al. Total hip arthroplasty performed without cement in patients with femoral head osteonecrosis who are less than 50 years old. J Arthroplasty 1998;13:876–81.

31. Hartley WT, McAuley JP, Culpepper WJ, et al. Osteonecrosis of the femoral head treated with cementless total hip arthroplasty. J Bone Joint Surg 2000;82-A:1408–13.

32. Xenakis TA, Gelalis J, Koukoubis TA, et al. Cementless hip arthroplasty in the treatment of patients with femoral head necrosis. Clin Orthop Relat Res 2001;386:93–9.

33. Fyda TM, Callaghan JJ, Olejniczak J, et al. Minimum ten-year follow-up of cemented total hip replacement in patients with osteonecrosis of the femoral head. Iowa Orthop J 2002;22:8–19.

34. Mont MA, Seyler TM, Plate JF, et al. Uncemented total hip arthroplasty in young adults with osteonecrosis of the femoral head: a comparative study. J Bone Joint Surg 2006;88(Suppl 3):104–9.

Total Hip Arthroplasty After Failed Treatment for Osteonecrosis of the Femoral Head

Wim HC. Rijnen, MD, Nanette Lameijn, MD,
B. Willem Schreurs, MD, PhD, Jean WM. Gardeniers, MD, PhD*

KEYWORDS
- Osteonecrosis • Hip • Total hip arthroplasty
- Avascular necrosis • Sugioka's osteotomy
- Bone impaction grafting

Osteonecrosis of the hip is a painful disorder mostly affecting young patients. Without specific treatment, osteonecrosis will lead to collapse of the femoral head and secondary osteoarthritis of the hip.[1] Femoral head-preserving treatments should slow down or even prevent the progress of collapse and degenerative changes. The goal is to postpone the final treatment with a total hip arthroplasty (THA) as long as possible. When earlier femoral head-preserving treatments fail, THA seems to be the final treatment of choice. This underscores the importance of femoral head-preserving procedures that not do hamper the technical procedure and outcome of a subsequent THA.

The transtrochanteric rotational osteotomy (TRO) for treatment of osteonecrosis of the femoral head was introduced by Sugioka[2] in 1972. This is a method in which the necrotic segment of the femoral head is rotated out of the weight-bearing area of the acetabulum. This is done after the greater trochanter is osteotomized and the medial circumflex femoral artery carefully preserved. An osteotomy is made perpendicular to the neck and the proximal femur is rotated around the axis of the femoral neck and fixated. In the authors' experience, with a mean follow-up of 8.7 years, 17 of 26 hips were converted to a THA. The clinical survival rate was 56% after 7 years and the radiologic survival rate was 54% after 1 year.[3] The promising clinical results achieved by Sugioka[4] (success rate 78% after 3–16 years of follow-up) cannot be matched by other surgeons. This is especially true for studies by European and American surgeons, who had disappointing results, mainly because of early osteoarthritis.[3,5–7]

Another femoral head-preserving treatment for osteonecrosis of the femoral head is the bone impaction grafting (BIG) technique. In this technique, a lateral approach is used as in a traditional core decompression. The osteonecrotic lesion inside the femoral head is removed and impacted bone grafts are used to regain stability and sphericity and to prevent collapse. In the authors' experience, a mean follow-up of 42 months, eight hips (29%) were converted to a THA. Of the 20 reconstructions that were in situ, 18 were clinically successful (90%) and 70% were radiologically successful.[8]

THAs performed after sub- or intertrochanteric osteotomies are known to have a higher rate of complications when compared with patients without previous osteotomy.[9–12] The perioperative and postoperative outcome of THA after a TRO according to Sugioka may be declined because of an anatomic deformity in the proximal femur after this osteotomy.

THA as a treatment modality in patients with osteonecrosis was initially associated with inferior long-term results.[13–20] Cemented THAs using the

---

Department of Orthopaedics, Radboud University Nijmegen Medical Centre, Post Box 9101, 6500 HB Nijmegen, The Netherlands
* Corresponding author.
E-mail address: J.Gardeniers@orthop.umcn.nl (J.WM. Gardeniers).

Orthop Clin N Am 40 (2009) 291–298
doi:10.1016/j.ocl.2009.01.001

latest generation cementing techniques and also hybrid and uncemented implants have improved these results remarkably.[21,22]

The purpose of this study was to evaluate the complications and the clinical and radiologic outcome of THA after failed TRO according to Sugioka (THA after TRO), and after failed BIG technique (THA after BIG) for osteonecrosis of the femoral head. The authors hypothesize that the BIG technique would lead to fewer complications and a better clinical outcome for a subsequent THA, compared with patients who underwent a TRO according to Sugioka before THA was performed.

MATERIALS AND METHODS
THA after TRO According to Sugioka

From September 1992 to February 1997, 26 consecutive hips in 22 patients with osteonecrosis of the femoral head were treated with TRO according to Sugioka. The age of the patients at time of the osteotomy was 30 years (range, 22–46 years). The original peri- and postoperative protocol by Sugioka was strictly followed, including the post-treatment protocol of nonweight bearing for 6 months. All operations were all performed by one surgeon (JWMG), who studied the technique in Japan by Sugioka.

After a mean follow-up time of 4.7 years (range, 1.4–10.1 years), a THA was performed on 17 hips from 14 patients after a failed TRO. One patient was lost to follow-up. The authors investigated 16 hip joints in 13 patients with a minimal follow-up of 2 years (**Table 1**). Before Sugioka's osteotomy was performed, the hips were graded for osteonecrosis using the staging system of the Association Research Circulation Osseous (ARCO).[23] However, according to Steinberg and colleagues,[24] Stage 3 was subdivided into "early" (without collapse of the femoral head) and "late" (with a collapse). Four hips were classified as Stage 2CC, one was Stage 3CC early, ten were Stage 3CC late, and one hip was classified as Stage 3CB late. The mean age at time of THA was 35 years (range, 24–53 years). The average follow-up after conversion to THA was 6.4 years (range 2.2–12.7 years).

The reason for conversion to a THA was a failure of the TRO because of culture-proven infection in two cases: one after the index surgery, the second after removal of screws because of pain in a consolidated osteotomy. In both cases this resulted in a resection arthroplasty despite debridement and treatment with antibiotics. After antibiotic treatment of the infection, both were successfully converted to a THA. In two cases

there was failure of the osteosynthesis material: in one patient a nonunion of the osteotomy 29 months after surgery. In 11 hips, a conversion into a THA was done because of symptoms relating to severe secondary osteoarthritis.

In one patient the osteosynthesis material was removed before THA was done. In all other patients it was done during the THA operation. Four patients underwent a re-operation before THA was performed; screws were changed for a dynamic hip screw in two patients and screws were changed for an angular plate in two other patients.

THA after BIG

Between 1992 and 2004, the authors performed BIG in 60 hips in patients with osteonecrosis of the femoral head. All operations were done by one surgeon (JWMG). The authors included all patients that underwent a THA after failed BIG for osteonecrosis of the femoral head, with a minimum follow-up of 2 years. From February 1999 to September 2004, THA was performed in 17 hips from 14 patients; no patient was lost to follow-up (see **Table 1**). Before BIG was performed, hips were graded according to the ARCO staging system, modified by Steinberg.[23,24] One hip was classified Stage 2BC, two were Stage 2CC, four were 3CC early, nine were 3CC late, and one hip was classified as Stage 3CB late.

The mean age at the time of the THA was 39 years (range, 25–49 years). THA was done at a mean follow-up time of 2.3 years (range, 0.5–5.7 years) after BIG was performed. The average follow-up after conversion into THA was 4.2 years (range, 2.1–7.3 years). The reason for conversion to a THA was because of complaints caused by pain from severe secondary osteoarthritis in all cases. No reoperations were performed between the BIG and the subsequent THA and no infections occurred.

All THAs that were performed were cemented total hips. The Exeter total hip system (Stryker, Newbury, U.K.) was used in all replacements, except in one where a Charnley Elite Plus total hip prosthesis (DePuy, Leeds, U.K.) was used.

The clinical follow-up of both groups of all patients consisted of the determination of preoperative and postoperative serial Harris Hip Scores (HHS),[25] and serial anterioposterior and lateral radiographs were used for the radiographic follow-up. The complication rate was determined; complications were defined as infection after THA, dislocation of THA, revision of THA for any reason, and radiologic loosening of THA. Valgus or varus stem malalignment was defined as deviation

Table 1
Patient characteristics

	Sugioka	BIG
Number of patients (hip joints)	13 (16)	14 (17)
Sex (male:female)	9:4	12:3
Affected side (right:left)	6:10	11:6
Cause of osteonecrosis		
Corticosteroids	9	9
Idiopathic	4	3
Alcohol	—	2
Posttraumatic	3	2
Hyperlipidemia	—	1
Body mass index	24 (20–33)	26 (19–35)
Age at time of Sugioka/BIG (years)	30 (22–46)	37 (24–46)
Age at time of THA (years)	35 (24–53)	39 (25–49)
Time interval Sugioka/BIG–THA (years)	4.7 (1.4–10.1)	2.3 (0.5–5.7)
Follow-up (years)	6.4 (2.2–12.7)	4.2 (2.1–7.3)

from the longitudinal femoral axis of more than 2 degrees measured on the anterioposterior radiographs.

Radiolucent lines of the femoral stem were allocated to Gruen regions 1 to 7.[26] A femoral stem was regarded loose if radiolucent lines greater than 2 mm were present around the entire implant. Radiolucency of the socket was assessed on the anterioposterior radiographs with the method of DeLee and Charnley,[27] with a radiolucent line measuring 2 mm in width considered as loosening of the cup. Heterotopic ossification was classified according to the system of Brooker and colleagues.[28]

Statistical Analysis

The generalized Wilcoxon test was used to test differences in progression between the groups for statistical significance. Fisher's Exact test was used to test differences between the groups for statistical significance in case of two-by-two tables. A P value of less than 0.05 was considered statistically significant.

Kaplan-Meier's survivorship analysis was used to assess the survival of the THA with revision of the acetabular of femoral component for any reason.

RESULTS

In the THA after TRO group, several difficulties were encountered during THA surgery. The original anatomy was grossly disturbed. The external rotators were completely unrecognizable in most cases. In two cases, locating of screws and cerclages was difficult. In another two cases, the screws could not be removed and the femoral head had to be resected into pieces before the screws could be taken out. In all conversions into THA, vast amounts of fibrous and connective tissue restricted a reasonable progress of surgery significantly. The proximal femur was anatomically highly distorted. The preplanned prosthesis could not be fitted in most cases.

No perioperative complications were observed in the THA after BIG group. After surgery, all patients followed a standard rehabilitation and training program as generally used for patients after a total hip arthroplasty.

The operating time in THA after TRO (median 158 minutes; 95% confidence interval or CI 136 186) was significantly longer ($P = .0042$, Wilcoxon test) than in THA after BIG (median 120 minutes; 95% CI 97–140). Perioperative blood loss in THA after TRO (median 1,350 cc; 95% CI 1050–1750) was significantly more ($P = .0014$, Wilcoxon test) than in THA after BIG (median 750 cc; 95% CI 535–950). Average hospital stay in THA after TRO was 11 days (range, 7–30 days), compared with an average of 9 days (range, 6–17 days) in THA after BIG ($P = .08$, Wilcoxon test) (**Table 2**).

In the postoperative phase, two patients in the THA after TRO group developed a culture-proven infection. The first patient developed an infection with a *Pseudomonas aeruginosa* 26 months after the index operation was performed and ended in a resection arthroplasty. This infection was treated with antibiotics and 8 months later, a new THA could be placed successfully. Another patient

Table 2
Clinical assessment of total hip arthroplasty after failed transtrochanteric rotational osteotomy according to Sugioka and after failed bone impaction grafting

	THA after Sugioka	THA after BIG	P
Blood loss (cc)	1,386 cc (400–2,600)	787 cc (180–2,500)	0.0014 (Wilcoxon test)
Operation time (minutes)	161 (15–235)	123 (70–188)	0.0042 (Wilcoxon test)
Hospital admission (days)	11 (7–30)	9 (6–17)	0.08 (Wilcoxon test)
Postoperative infections	2	0	0.2273 (Fisher's exact test)
Postoperative luxations	2	0	0.2273 (Fisher's exact test)
HHS preoperative	52 (28–81)	42 (16–69)	0.06 (Wilcoxon test)
HHS postoperative	89 (53–100)	91 (40–100)	0.94 (Wilcoxon test)

developed an infection with a methicillin-resistant *Staphylococcus epidermidis* 3 months after the index operation. This was initially treated with debridement and treatment with antibiotics. However, 6 years after the THA was performed, the infection recurred and the THA had to be removed. Twenty months later a new THA was performed. In the THA after BIG group, no infections occurred.

In the THA after TRO group, two patients had dislocations of the THA. One patient underwent surgery for refixation of the greater trochanter after two dislocations. The other patient underwent revision of the THA 3 years after the initial THA was performed. In the THA after BIG group, no dislocations occurred.

In the THA after BIG group, in one case, revision of the socket was performed 28 months after placement because of aseptic loosening.

The overall average HHS for the group before THA after TRO was 52 points (range, 28–81 points), which improved to 89 points (range, 53–100 points) at final follow-up. The average HHS for the group before THA after BIG was 42 (range, 16–69 points), which improved to 91 points (range, 40–100 points) at final follow-up.

The increase of HHS per year is significantly higher for the group THA after BIG compared with the group THA after TRO ($P = .0004$). After excluding the failures resulting from infection or revision for any reason, the mean HHS for the group THA after TRO was 50 points (range, 28–68 points), which improved to 93 points (range, 73–100 points) at final follow-up. The mean HHS for the group before THA after BIG was 43 (range, 16–69 points), which improved to 94 points (range, 83–100 points) at final follow-up.

Kaplan-Meier analysis, with revision of THA for any reason as endpoint (**Fig. 1**), shows a decline in survival for the THA after TRO group.

The overall complication rate for the THA after the Sugioka group is 31% (5 out of 16). The complication rate for the THA after BIG group is 6% (1 out of 17). After excluding the two patients with infections, the overall complication rate for the THA after Sugioka group is 19% (3 out of 16).

Radiology

In the THA after TRO group, the position of the femoral prosthesis was neutral in three hips, ten hips had a varus position (**Fig. 2**), and three hips had a valgus position. In the THA after BIG group, the position of the femoral prosthesis was neutral in eight hips, eight hips had a varus position, and one hip had a valgus position. In the THA after TRO group, five hips had more than 4 degrees of malalignment, compared with three hips in the THA after BIG group.

In the THA after TRO group, in one patient a radiographic loosening of the socket was observed. In this case there was also accompanying radiolucency in Gruen zones 2 and 3 of the stem 26 months after THA placement. At time of follow-up, no revision of this THA was performed.

In the THA after TRO group, in two hips there was radiolucency in zone 1 of the socket without signs of radiographic loosening. This was also observed in one hip of the THA after BIG group. In the THA after TRO group, subsidence of the stem of 1 mm was observed in three hips and broken cerclage wires of the major trochanter in two hips. In both groups, a periarticular ossification was observed in one hip, a Brooker grade 1 in the THA after BIG group, and a Brooker grade 2 in the THA after TRO group.

DISCUSSION

The purpose of this study was to evaluate the complications and the clinical and radiologic

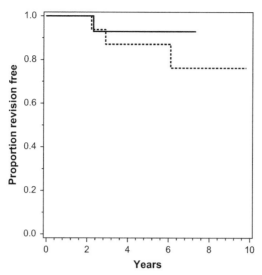

Fig. 1. Kaplan-Meier survivorship curves for total hip arthroplasty after failed BIG (*dashed line*) and after failed TRO according to Sugioka (*dotted line*), with revision of the acetabular of femoral component for any reason as endpoint. (*P* = .17, Mantel-Cox log-rank test).

outcome of THA after failed TRO according to Sugioka (THA after TRO) and after failed BIG technique (THA after BIG) for osteonecrosis of the femoral head. THA after TRO compared with THA after BIG led to a higher complication rate; that is, the rate of revision THA for any reason, radiologic loosening of the THA, infections, and dislocations, was higher. This led to a complication rate of 31% in the THA after Sugioka group, compared with only 6% for the THA after BIG group. Furthermore, in the THA after Sugioka group, operation time was longer, there was more perioperative blood loss, and the duration of hospital admission was longer compared with the THA after BIG group. However, because of the relatively low number of patients and a midterm follow-up period, the survival was not significantly different.

Sugioka's osteotomy is a technically highly demanding procedure with disappointing results in non-Japanese studies.[5–7] The authors described their experience with this osteotomy

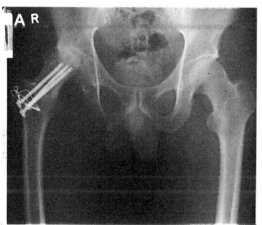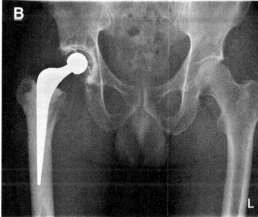

Fig. 2. (*A*) X-ray of a patient who underwent a TRO according to Sugioka because of a noncollapsed osteonecrosis of the femoral head. The reason for conversion into a total hip arthroplasty 36 months after the osteotomy was because of complaints of progressive secondary osteoarthritis with a Harris Hip Score of 53 and major restrictions in the range of motion of the hip joint. (*B*) X-ray of the same patient 10 years after total hip arthroplasty was performed. The stem is positioned in a 6 degrees varus malalignment.

earlier,[3] and the high rate of problems with osteosynthesis, infections, and the inability to delay the osteoarthritic process effectively. Revision into a THA after a failed TRO according to Sugioka is a challenging procedure.

Different studies describe the outcome of THA after an osteotomy of the proximal femur. The report of Kawasaki and colleagues[11] is the only study that describes the outcome of hips that were converted to a THA after a failed TRO. Their complication rate was 26%, but they concluded that the osteotomy did not influence the outcome of a secondary THA. They do describe a significantly longer operation time in the THA after TRO group and significantly more blood loss in the THA after TRO group, compared with a matched control group with primary THA for osteonecrosis of the femoral head. The technical difficulties were mainly because of the rotational change in the geometry of the proximal part of the femur. In the authors' study, varus malalignment of the femoral prosthesis was observed, mainly in the THA after TRO group. This was caused by the deformity of the proximal femur after the osteotomy and the progressive varus deformity of the neck of the femur that could be observed in some patients.

Boos and colleagues[9] stated that THA after previous intertrochanteric osteotomy is technically more demanding with a longer operating time, but not necessarily associated with a higher rate of complications. There was, however, a trend toward improved survival in the group without previous osteotomy. Ferguson and colleagues[10] report technical failures at operation in 23% and a total perioperative complication rate of 11.8% in patients who received a THA after failed intertrochanteric osteotomy.

Soballe and colleagues[29] concluded that when an intertrochanteric osteotomy is only slightly displaced, it can be used to treat osteoarthritis without sacrificing the quality of a subsequent cemented total hip replacement. This correlates with the study of Breusch and colleagues,[30] who found similar outcome of uncemented THA after intertrochanteric osteotomy and patients with regular femoral anatomy. Shinar and Harris[12] stated that intertrochanteric osteotomy, in general, did not affect the expected excellent results of the femoral component using modern cementation techniques. Severe deformity following subtrochanteric osteotomy, however, did adversely affect the outcome. Haverkamp and colleagues[31] suggest the long term-term outcome of a cemented THA is not impaired by a previous well-performed osteotomy. In their article, they give a clear overview and comparison of the available literature about this topic.

Iwase and colleagues[32] compared cemented and uncemented THA after intertrochanteric osteotomy of the proximal femur and found that survivorship of cemented stems was significantly higher than that of conventional cementless stems.

The BIG technique is a salvage procedure developed for osteonecrosis of the femoral head.[8] At midterm, follow-up results were promising. Furthermore, in the authors' opinion, the procedure does not intervene with revision into a THA afterwards. This is confirmed by Rosenwasser and colleagues,[33] who did not find technical difficulties while performing THA after cancellous bone grafting using the lightbulb procedure for osteonecrosis of the femoral head. Mont and colleagues[34] used the trapdoor procedure using cortical and cancellous bone grafts for treatment of osteonecrosis of the femoral head. In the patients who required conversion into THA, procedures were performed without complications related to the previous trapdoor procedure.

THA as treatment modality in patients with osteonecrosis was initially associated with inferior long-term results. Different causes are mentioned, including the relative youth of patients, their long life expectancy, the inferior quality of bone with different tissue response, and persistent defects in bone mineral metabolism.[13,15–18] Especially when performed in hips with advanced stages of osteonecrosis and in patients under 30 years old, total hip replacement showed universally bad results.[14,19,20] Failure rates were four times higher than the same procedure performed in osteoarthritic hips.[20] The latest generation cementing technique and hybrid and uncemented components have improved on these early results.[21,22]

In the authors' opinion, the higher rate of complications and revision of THA in the THA after TRO group was caused by the disturbed anatomy after the TRO. In the THA after BIG group, the initial anatomy is not disturbed as after an osteotomy.

SUMMARY

Results are presented for THA after failed TRO (THA after TRO) according to Sugioka and after failed BIG (THA after BIG), both initially performed for osteonecrosis of the femoral head. After a minimal follow-up of 2 years, 33 hips were studied. In THA after TRO when compared with THA after BIG, clinical and radiologic outcome was less favorable, more complications were observed, and there was a higher revision rate in a technically more demanding procedure.

REFERENCES

1. Musso ES, Mitchell SN, Schink-Ascani M, et al. Results of conservative management of osteonecrosis of the femoral head. A retrospective review. Clin Orthop Relat Res 1986;207:209–15.

2. Sugioka Y. Transtrochanteric anterior rotational osteotomy of the femoral head in the treatment of osteonecrosis affecting the hip: a new osteotomy operation. Clin Orthop Relat Res 1978;130:191–201.

3. Rijnen WH, Gardeniers JW, Westrek BL, et al. Sugioka's osteotomy for femoral-head necrosis in young Caucasians. Int Orthop 2005;9:140–4.

4. Sugioka Y, Hotokebuchi T, Tsutsui H. Transtrochanteric anterior rotational osteotomy for idiopathic and steroid-induced necrosis of the femoral head: indications and long-term results. Clin Orthop Relat Res 1992;277:111–20.

5. Dean MT, Cabanela ME. Transtrochanteric anterior rotational osteotomy for avascular necrosis of the femoral head: long-term results. J Bone Joint Surg Br 1993;75:597–601.

6. Langlais F, Fourastier J. Rotation osteotomies for osteonecrosis of the femoral head. Clin Orthop Relat Res 1997;343:110–23.

7. Tooke SMT, Amstutz HC, Hedley AK. Results of transtrochanteric rotational osteotomy for femoral head osteonecrosis. Clin Orthop Relat Res 1987;224:150–7.

8. Rijnen WH, Gardeniers JW, Buma P, et al. Treatment of femoral head osteonecrosis using bone impaction grafting. Clin Orthop Relat Res 2003;417:74–83.

9. Boos N, Krushell R, Ganz R, et al. Total hip arthroplasty after previous proximal femoral osteotomy. J Bone Joint Surg Br 1997;79(2):247–53.

10. Ferguson GM, Cabanela ME, Ilstrup DM. Total hip arthroplasty after failed intertrochanteric osteotomy. J Bone Joint Surg Br 1994;76(2):252–7.

11. Kawasaki M, Hasegawa Y, Sakano S, et al. Total hip arthoplasty after failed transtrochanteric rotational osteotomy for avascular necrosis of the femoral head. J Arthroplasty 2005;20(5):574–9.

12. Shinar AA, Harris WH. Cemented total hip arthroplasty following previous femoral osteotomy: an average 16-year follow-up study. J Arthroplasty 1998;13(3):243–53.

13. Calder JD, Pearse MF, Revell PA. The extent of osteocyte death in the proximal femur of patients with osteonecrosis of the femoral head. J Bone Joint Surg Br 2001;83(3):419–22.

14. Chandler HP, Reineck FT, Wixson RL, et al. Total hip replacement in patients younger than thirty years old. A five-year follow-up study. J Bone Joint Surg Am 1981;63(9):1426–34.

15. Cornell CN, Salvati EA, Pellicci PM. Long-term follow-up of total hip replacement in patients with osteonecrosis. Orthop Clin North Am 1985;16(4):757–69.

16. Dorr LD, Takei GK, Conaty JP. Total hip arthroplasties in patients less than forty-five years old. J Bone Joint Surg Am 1983;65(4):474–9.

17. Frassica FL, Berry DJ, Morrey BF. Avascular necrosis. In: Morrey BF, editor. Joint replacement arthroplasty. 3rd edition. Philadelphia: Churchill-Livingstone; 2003. p. 752–69.

18. Mont MA, Hungerford DS. Non-traumatic avascular necrosis of the femoral head. J Bone Joint Surg Am 1995;77(3):459–74.

19. Saito S, Saito M, Nishina T, et al. Long-term results of total hip arthroplasty for osteonecrosis of the femoral head. A comparison with osteoarthritis. Clin Orthop Relat Res 1989;244:198–207.

20. Salvati EA, Cornell CN. Long-term follow-up of total hip replacement in patients with avascular necrosis. Instr Course Lect 1988;37:67–73.

21. Garino JP, Steinberg ME. Total hip arthroplasty in patients with avascular necrosis of the femoral head: a 2- to 10-year follow-up. Clin Orthop Relat Res 1997;334:108–15.

22. Kim YH, Oh SH, Kim JS, et al. Contemporary total hip arthroplasty with and without cement in patients with osteonecrosis of the femoral head. J Bone Joint Surg Am 2003;85(4):675–81.

23. Gardeniers JWM, et al. The ARCO perspective for reaching one uniform staging system of osteonecrosis. In: Schoutens A, Arlet J, Gardeniers JWM, et al, editors. Bone circulation and vascularization in normal and pathological conditions. New York: Plenum Press; 1993. p. 375–80.

24. Steinberg ME, Haykan GD, Steinberg DR. A quantitative system for staging avascular necrosis. J Bone Joint Surg Br 1995;77:34–41.

25. Harris WH. Traumatic arthritis of the hip after dislocation and acetabular fractures: treatment by mold arthroplasty: An end-result study using a new method of result evaluation. J Bone Joint Surg Am 1969;51:737–55.

26. Gruen TA, McNeice GM, Amstutz HC. Modes of failure of cemented stem-type femoral components: a radiographic analysis of loosening. Clin Orthop Relat Res 1979;141:17–27.

27. DeLee JG, Charnley J. Radiological demarcation of cemented sockets in total hip replacement. Clin Orthop Relat Res 1976;121:20–32.

28. Brooker AF, Bowerman JW, Robinson RA, et al. Ectopic ossification following total hip replacement. Incidence and a method of classification. J Bone Joint Surg Am 1973;55:1629–32.

29. Soballe K, Boll KL, Kofod S, et al. Total hip replacement after medial-displacement osteotomy of the proximal part of the femur. J Bone Joint Surg Am 1989;71(5):692–7.

30. Breusch SJ, Lukoschek M, Thomsen M, et al. Ten-year results of uncemented hip stems for failed

intertrochanteric osteotomy. Arch Orthop Trauma Surg 2005;125(5):304–9.

31. Haverkamp D, De Jong PT, Marti RK. Introchanteric osteotomies do not impair long-term outcome of subsuquent cemented total hip arthroplasties. Clin Orthop Relat Res 2006;444:154–60.

32. Iwase T, Hasegawa Y, Iwasada S, et al. Total hip arthroplasty after failed intertrochanteric valgus osteotomy for advanced osteoarthrosis. Clin Orthop Relat Res 1999;364:175–81.

33. Rosenwasser MP, Garino JP, Kiernan HA, et al. Long term follow-up of thorough debridement and cancellous bone grafting of the femora head for avascular necrosis. Clin Orthop Relat Res 1994;306:17–27.

34. Mont MA, Einhorn TA, Sponseller PD, et al. The trapdoor procedure using autogenous and cancellous bone grafts for osteonecrosis of the femoral head. J Bone Joint Surg Br 1998;80 56–62.

Current Literature: An Educational Tool to Study Osteonecrosis for the Orthopaedic In-Training Examination?

David R. Marker, BS[a],*, Michael A. Mont, MD[b], Thorsten M. Seyler, MD[c],
Dawn M. LaPorte, MD[a], Frank J. Frassica, MD[a]

KEYWORDS

- Orthopaedic in-training examination
- Education • Osteonecrosis • Resident training
- Current literature

The Accreditation Council for Graduate Medical Education has defined *medical knowledge* as one of six clinical care domains in which residents must receive instruction and show competency.[1] The orthopedic community has long been a leader in this domain. In the 1960s, the American Academy of Orthopaedic Surgeons established the Orthopaedic In-Training Examination (OITE) as the first standard test used by a specialty to assess residents' medical knowledge.[2] This examination, developed to measure orthopedic resident education and knowledge, focuses on relevant information supported by current scientific literature. Because of this focus, recent publications are frequently used as an educational tool in nearly all residency programs.[3] In addition, recent reports say performance on the OITE directly correlates with frequent review of recent literature.[4]

Many studies in the current scientific literature focus on novel surgical techniques and management protocols that are limited to small study cohorts, have limited follow-up, or are controversial. For example, although our understanding of osteonecrosis has advanced, the pathogenesis, associated risk factors, and diagnosis of osteonecrosis are still not fully understood.[5–8] In addition, the treatment of osteonecrosis remains controversial with management ranging from non-operative modalities[9] and pharmacologics[10,11] to more invasive procedures, such as core decompression[12,13] and total joint arthroplasty.[14,15] Based on this lack of consensus regarding the management of such diseases as osteonecrosis, the relevance of current literature as a study tool for the OITE is unclear. This uncertainty was one of the justifications for this study.

The purpose of the present study was to assess the relevance of recent literature as a tool for young physicians learning more about osteonecrosis as they prepare for the OITE and their future board certification. The three primary questions we asked were:

What is the character of the osteonecrosis questions on the OITE?
What are the recommended references for the OITE questions?
Do the osteonecrosis-related questions correlate with the current literature?

While this study focused on osteonecrosis-related material on the OITE, we also looked at other subject areas frequently tested on the OITE

[a] Johns Hopkins University School of Medicine, 601 North Caroline Street, Baltimore, MD 21287, USA
[b] Rubin Institute for Advanced Orthopedics, Center for Joint Preservation and Reconstruction, Sinai Hospital of Baltimore, 2401 West Belvedere Avenue, Baltimore, MD 21215, USA
[c] Department of Orthopaedic Surgery, Wake Forest University School of Medicine, Medical Center Boulevard, Winston-Salem, NC 27157, USA
* Corresponding author.
E-mail address: dmarker2@jhmi.edu (D.R. Marker).

Orthop Clin N Am 40 (2009) 299–304
doi:10.1016/j.ocl.2008.10.011

to further assess the relevance of recent literature as a study tool.

METHODS

A systematic review was conducted of the OITE to identify all osteonecrosis-related questions tested during a 5-year period (2002–2006). The questions were stratified according to four subject areas: etiology/associated risk factors, pathology/pathophysiology, diagnosis/classification, and treatment. Questions related to the treatment of osteonecrosis were further stratified according to the following subcategories: noninvasive (such as pharmacologic treatment and shock-wave treatment), core decompressions and nonvascularized graftings, revascularization techniques, osteotomies, and replacement surgeries (such as total hip arthroplasty and hemi- and total hip resurfacing).

For each of the osteonecrosis-related questions, the recommended readings were reviewed and the most frequently referenced journals and textbooks were identified. These recommended references are provided as part of the OITE score key distributed by the American Academy of Orthopaedic Surgeons. Each question has one or more references recommended for the test material.

Next, a systematic review was conducted using the Medline bibliographic databases of all literature from the 5 years that preceded the OITE (2001–2005) in four high-impact orthopedic journals (a total of 6750 articles): *The Journal of Bone and Joint Surgery American*, *Clinical Orthopaedics and Related Research*, *Journal of Arthroplasty*, and *Journal of Orthopaedic Research*. For each year, the total number of articles and the number of articles related to osteonecrosis or avascular necrosis were determined. All articles were screened by two reviewers and grouped as having either a primary or secondary focus on osteonecrosis. An example of an article grouped as having a secondary focus is one that reports on mortality following shoulder arthroplasty with the reason for surgery being osteonecrosis in only 1 of 17 patients.[16] The primary-focus articles were stratified in a similar manner as that for the OITE questions.

To further assess the current literature as a tool for preparing for the OITE, a similar analysis was also conducted for four other subject areas tested on the OITE: idiopathic scoliosis, chondrosarcoma, femoral neck fracture, and hip resurfacing. As with the osteonecrosis OITE questions, the questions for these subject areas were screened and grouped as having either a primary or secondary focus and

then stratified by subcategories. As many as five of the following relevant journals were reviewed for each subject area: *The Journal of Bone and Joint Surgery American*, *Clinical Orthopaedics and Related Research*, *Journal of Arthroplasty*, *Journal of Orthopaedic Research*, *Spine*, and *Journal of Pediatric Orthopaedics*.

All data were subjected to averaging and analysis using SPSS (Statistical Package for the Social Sciences) v13.0 software (SPSS, Chicago, Illinois). The overall proportions and the percentages in each category were compared between the OITE questions and the literature. The difference in proportions was assessed using a chi-square analysis with Yate's correction, where a P value of less than .05 was considered significant.

RESULTS

Overall, 0.6% (range, 0%–1%) of the OITE questions had a primary osteonecrosis focus. The most common category of question tested was diagnosis and classification of osteonecrosis. No questions were related to the pathology of the disease. While 25% of the questions required knowledge concerning the treatment of osteonecrosis, there were no questions regarding various treatments, such as core decompression, pharmacologic treatment, core decompressions, nonvascularized graftings, revascularization techniques, and osteotomies. Total joint arthroplasty was the only treatment subcategory tested on the OITE.

The review of the recommended references for the OITE osteonecrosis-related questions showed that 72% were journal articles and 28% were textbooks. For all of the questions, more than one recommended reference was provided. *The Journal of Bone and Joint Surgery American* and *Clinical Orthopaedics and Related Research* were the two most cited references, and together they represented 33% of all of the references.

One hundred thirty-six (2.0%) of the studies in the reviewed current literature were classified as having a primary focus on osteonecrosis while 115 (1.7%) had a secondary focus on osteonecrosis. There were 30 primary-focus articles every year except for 2002 when there were 16. Out of the four journals reviewed, *Clinical Orthopaedics and Related Research* had the highest percentage of etiology–and risk-factor–related articles (25%), whereas *Journal of Orthopaedic Research* was the most concentrated in pathology (33%) and diagnosis/classification (33%). *Journal of Arthroplasty* articles were mostly focused on treatment (83%). The percentage of OITE questions (0.6%) that had a primary osteonecrosis focus was statistically lower than the overall percentage of osteonecrosis articles (2.0%) (P<.001). Similarly, the percentage was consistently lower during each of the 5 years reviewed (**Fig. 1**). The percentage of OITE questions (50%) classified as related to diagnosis and classification of osteonecrosis was higher that the proportion of articles (11%) in the journals reviewed (P = .005). Grouped by treatment, etiology/risk factors, and pathology, there were, respectively, 55%, 22%, and 12% for the articles compared with 25%, 25%, and 0% for the OITE questions. Because of the relatively small numbers of OITE questions, none of these differences was determined to be statistically significant. As previously noted, total joint arthroplasty was the only treatment subcategory tested on the OITE. In contrast, more than half of the articles that discussed the treatment of osteonecrosis reported modalities other than total joint arthroplasty (**Fig. 2**).

The average percentage of articles related to idiopathic scoliosis, chondrosarcoma, femoral neck fracture, and hip resurfacing were 2.6% (range, 0.2%–7.2%), 0.5% (range, 0.3%–1.2%), 0.7% (range, 0.2%–1.6%), and 0.3% (range, 0%–0.6%), respectively. The corresponding percentages for the OITE were, respectively, 0.7%, 0.6%, 0.6%, and 0.3% for the same subject areas. The OITE reflected the change in the number of articles in some subjects. For example, the increase in resurfacing articles from 0.17% in 2001 to 0.58% in 2005 corresponded to an increase from 0% to 0.73% in the corresponding number of OITE questions related to resurfacing arthroplasty (**Table 1**). However, for other subject matter, there was a significant difference between the literature

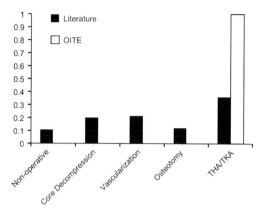

Fig. 2. Proportion for the subcategories for treatment of osteonecrosis on the OITE versus that for the same subcategories in the reviewed current literature. THA/TKA, total hip arthroplasty/total knee arthroplasty.

and the examination. For example, the year with the most articles about femoral neck fractures (2002 with 1.3%) was followed by an OITE that had no primary-focus questions about this subject.

SUMMARY

The OITE is a standardized test developed by the American Academy of Orthopaedic Surgeons in the 1960s as the first standard test used by a specialty to assess residents' medical knowledge.[2] The examination is designed to test resident knowledge regarding pathology, diagnosis, and treatment of orthopedic diseases based on the current scientific literature. Many orthopedic residents study the current literature and journal clubs are commonly used by orthopedic programs as a teaching modality.[3,17] However, at the time of this study, no studies to the authors' knowledge had assessed the correlation between the literature and the content tested on the examination. This study assessed the relevance of current literature as a study tool for the OITE, especially for osteonecrosis.

One of the purposes of this study was to characterize the osteonecrosis-related content tested on the OITE. The concept of analyzing the content and type of questions on the OITE was first proposed in the literature in a study by Frassica and colleagues.[18] Their study focused on the core of pathology knowledge required on the OITE. They reported that approximately 10% of the examination is composed of pathology-related questions. Stratification of these questions showed that the majority of the questions required the resident to interpret imaging studies alone or imaging studies and histologic material. The

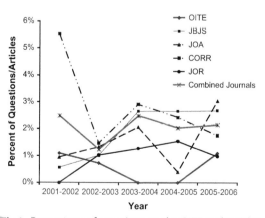

Fig. 1. Percentage of questions on the OITE and articles in the journals reviewed over a 5-year period. CORR, *Clinical Orthopaedics and Related Research*; JBJS, *The Journal of Bone and Joint Surgery American*; JOA, *Journal of Arthroplasty*; JOR, *Journal of Orthopaedic Research*.

Table 1
Comparison of the content on the Orthopaedic In-Training Examination versus that of current literature

	Content Topic				
Period	Osteonecrosis	Femoral Neck Fracture	Hip Resurfacing	Chondrosarcoma	Scoliosis
2001–2002					
Literature	2.49%	0.26%	0.17%	0.63%	2.40%
OITE	1.09%	0.36%	0.00%	0.73%	1.45%
2002–2003					
Literature	1.24%	1.46%	0.08%	0.79%	2.77%
OITE	0.73%	0.00%	0.36%	0.73%	0.73%
2003–2004					
Literature	2.14%	0.80%	0.14%	0.46%	2.44%
OITE	0.00%	1.09%	0.36%	0.73%	0.36%
2004–2005					
Literature	2.04%	0.50%	0.48%	0.45%	2.30%
OITE	0.00%	0.36%	0.00%	0.73%	0.00%
2005–2006					
Literature	2.16%	0.60%	0.58%	0.22%	2.91%
OITE	1.09%	1.09%	0.73%	0.00%	0.73%
Total					
Literature	2.01%	0.72%	0.30%	0.51%	2.57%[a]
OITE	0.58%	0.58%	0.30%	0.58%	0.65%
P value	<.001[b]	.700	.787	.961	<.001[b]

[a] If the articles reviewed from the specialty journal for this subcategory (*Spine*) were excluded, the percent of literature articles was 0.45%; and there was no statistical difference between the OITE and literature.
[b] Statistically significant.

results of the present study were similar and suggest that residents preparing for osteonecrosis-related questions on the OITE would benefit most by studying those articles related to the diagnosis and classification of the disease.

In each of the journals reviewed for this study, the percentage of articles focused on osteonecrosis was greater than the percentage of OITE questions focused on osteonecrosis. There are a number of possible explanations for this discrepancy. Although osteonecrosis is a debilitating disease, it does not present as a life-threatening illness. So the potential consequences of failing to recognize the illness are not as harmful as those for missing more catastrophic diseases. It is appropriate that the OITE emphasize disease processes that, if missed by the practicing orthopedic surgeon, could lead to serious morbidity to the patient or even mortality. With respect to the difference in emphasis between the material tested on the OITE and that in the literature, the OITE focused more on diagnosis and the only treatment modality tested in a question was total joint arthroplasty (**Fig. 3**). This difference can likely be attributed to the fact that total joint arthroplasty is generally accepted as the recommended treatment for late-stage disease. For early-stage disease, opinion remains divided. For example, a recent article by Hungerford[13] suggests that such procedures as vascularized bone grafting and femoral osteotomy, which have a low success rate, high complication rate, and high morbidity, and procedures that compromise subsequent total hip arthroplasty should not be recommended. However, other investigators continue to report the effective use of these treatment modalities.[19,20] These conflicting reports emphasize the need for more prospective, randomized studies and multi-center collaboration to better define the appropriate treatment for early-stage osteonecrosis.

Overall, the OITE and the literature had similar proportions of questions and articles for a number of the subject areas and subcategories reviewed. This suggests that current literature can be a useful study tool for the OITE. This recommendation is further strengthened by the results of a recent study, by Miyamoto and colleagues,[4] that reported a direct correlation between performance on the OITE and the use of specific current orthopedic literature and other relevant study habits. They

---

Osteonecrosis-related question similar to the OITE

What is the most appropriate treatment for a patient who has end stage osteonecrosis of the humeral head with glenoid degeneration?

    A. Core decompression

    B. Bipolar hemiarthroplasty

    C. Total shoulder arthroplasty

    D. Tantalum screw

    E. Vascularized fibular autografting

(Answer: C. Total shoulder arthroplasty)

Fig. 3. A hypothetical question similar to questions on the OITE testing osteonecrosis-related knowledge.

showed that reporting use by residents of both the *Journal of Bone and Joint Surgery American* and the *Journal of the American Academy of Orthopaedic Surgeons* had coefficients of 0.6 ($P<.01$) and 0.36 ($P = .02$) respectively for correlation with OITE performance. Other factors shown to have a positive correlation with performance were use of prior OITEs (correlation coefficient for bivariate analysis [r] = 0.53, $P<.001$), use of self-assessment examinations (r = 0.64, $P<.001$), daily orthopedic reading (r = 0.34, $P = .03$), increased preparation time for OITE (r = 0.31, $P = .04$), and more hours committed to studying (r = 0.37, $P = .01$).

Our study showed some discrepancies between the journals and the examination for certain subject areas, such as idiopathic scoliosis and osteonecrosis. These differences may be due to the emphasis of some of the journals on a specific subject area or on nonvalidated procedures. For example, there was a statistical difference in the total proportion of articles versus questions related to idiopathic scoliosis (2.57% versus 0.65%, $P<.001$). However, further examination showed that when excluding the subspecialty journal reviewed for idiopathic scoliosis, which had 7% of its articles related to this topic, there was no statistical difference. These results suggest that residents preparing for the OITE would benefit by focusing on core journals rather than on subspecialty journals.

This study was limited to the review of orthopedic journals. However, journals from other specialty areas, such as rheumatology, may also include review material related to osteonecrosis. Such journals, broadly speaking, have marginal value in OITE preparation, but residents may still find them useful for understanding specific subject areas in greater detail. This study did not specifically assess the content of these journals.

The study of the current literature should become a practice that residents learn and take with them into their professional careers. While this study suggests that some publications may be less relevant than others for OITE preparation, the current literature does in part reflect the content of the examination. We recommend the current literature as an educational tool for orthopedic surgeons-in-training, but they should recognize that some studies, especially those assessing new techniques or protocols that are not yet widely adopted, are not likely to represent what will be tested. With an understanding of both the material tested on the OITE and the content of recent publications, academic orthopaedic surgeons can develop appropriate educational programs for their residents in training.

REFERENCES

1. Accreditation Council for Graduate Medical Education, Program requirements for graduate medical education in orthopaedics. Available at: http://www.acgme.org/acWebsite/downloads/RRC_progReq/260orthopaedicsurgery07012007.pdf. Accessed June 20, 2008.
2. Mankin HJ. The Orthopaedic In-Training Examination (OITE). Clin Orthop Relat Res 1971;75:108–16.
3. Greene WB. The role of journal clubs in orthopaedic surgery residency programs. Clin Orthop Relat Res 2000;373:304–10.
4. Miyamoto RG Jr, Klein GR, Walsh M, et al. Orthopedic surgery residents' study habits and performance

on the orthopedic in-training examination. Am J Orthop 2007;36:E185–8.

5. Min BW, Song KS, Cho CH, et al. Untreated asymptomatic hips in patients with osteonecrosis of the femoral head. Clin Orthop Relat Res 2008;466: 1087–92.

6. Bastian JD, Hertel R. Initial post-fracture humeral head ischemia does not predict development of necrosis. J Shoulder Elbow Surg 2008;17:2–8.

7. Mont MA, Ulrich SD, Hungerford DS, et al. Bone scanning of limited value for the diagnosis of symptomatic oligofocal and multifocal osteonecrosis. J Rheumatol 2008;35(8):1629–34.

8. Mont MA, Jones LC, Hungerford DS. Nontraumatic osteonecrosis of the femoral head: ten years later. J Bone Joint Surg Am 2006;88:1117–32.

9. Massari L, Fini M, Cadossi R, et al. Biophysical stimulation with pulsed electromagnetic fields in osteonecrosis of the femoral head. J Bone Joint Surg Am 2006;88(Suppl 3):56–60.

10. Nishida K, Yamamoto T, Motomura G, et al. Pitavastatin may reduce risk of steroid-induced osteonecrosis in rabbits: a preliminary histological study. Clin Orthop Relat Res 2008;466:1054–8.

11. Agarwala S, Jain D, Joshi VR, et al. Efficacy of alendronate, a bisphosphonate, in the treatment of AVN of the hip. A prospective open-label study. Rheumatology (Oxford) 2005;44:352–9.

12. Marker DR, Seyler TM, Ulrich SD, et al. Do modern techniques improve core decompression outcomes for hip osteonecrosis? Clin Orthop Relat Res 2008; 466:1093–103.

13. Hungerford DS. Treatment of osteonecrosis of the femoral head: everything's new. J Arthroplasty 2007;22:91–4.

14. Bailie DS, Llinas PJ, Ellenbecker TS. Cementless humeral resurfacing arthroplasty in active patients less than fifty-five years of age. J Bone Joint Surg Am 2008;90:110–7.

15. McGrory BJ, York SC, Iorio R, et al. Current practices of AAHKS members in the treatment of adult osteonecrosis of the femoral head. J Bone Joint Surg Am 2007;89:1194–204.

16. White CB, Sperling JW, Cofield RH, et al. Ninety-day mortality after shoulder arthroplasty. J Arthroplasty 2003;18:886–8.

17. Dirschl DR, Tornetta P 3rd, Bhandari M. Designing, conducting, and evaluating journal clubs in orthopaedic surgery. Clin Orthop Relat Res 2003;146–57.

18. Frassica FJ, Papp D, McCarthy E, et al. Analysis of the pathology section of the OITE will aid in trainee preparation. Clin Orthop Relat Res 2008;466:1323–8.

19. Aldridge JM 3rd, Urbaniak JR. Vascularized fibular grafting for osteonecrosis of the femoral head with unusual indications. Clin Orthop Relat Res 2008; 466:1117–24.

20. Yoon TR, Abbas AA, Hur CI, et al. Modified transtrochanteric rotational osteotomy for femoral head osteonecrosis. Clin Orthop Relat Res 2008;466: 1110–6.

Index

Note: Page numbers of article titles are in **boldface** type.

A

Accreditation Council for Graduate Medical Education, 299
Age, as factor in osteonecrosis of femoral head, 267
Arthroplasty
  for postarthroscopic osteonecrosis of the knee, 207–209
  hemi-resurfacing, for osteonecrosis of hip, 27–year experience with, **275–282.** See also *Hip(s), osteonecrosis of, hemi-resurfacing arthroplasty for, 27-year experience with.*
  total hip, after failed treatment for osteonecrosis of femoral head, study of, **291–298.** See also *Total hip arthroplasty (THA), after failed treatment for osteonecrosis of femoral head, study of.*
  total knee
    for secondary osteonecrosis of the knee, 206
    for SPONK, 202
  unilateral knee, for SPONK, 201–202
Arthroscopy
  core depression with, for secondary osteonecrosis of the knee, 205
  for SPONK, 199–200
Avascular necrosis, pathophysiology of, 249

B

Basic multicellular unit (BMU), 213
BIG. See *Bone impaction grafting (BIG).*
Biologic assessment, in osteonecrosis treatment evaluation, 185–187
Biologic improvement, clinical improvement vs., in osteonecrosis treatment, 179
Biomarkers, in osteonecrosis treatment evaluation, 187
Bisphosphonate(s)
  BRONJ due to, 228–231. See also *Bisphosphonate-related osteonecrosis of jaws (BRONJ).*
  contraindications to, 225
  FDA-approved, 225
  for osteonecrosis of femoral head, 226–228
  mechanism of action of, 224
  osteonecrosis and, **223–234**
  physiologic effects of, 224–225
  potency of, 224
  side effects of, 225–226
  structure of, 223
  uses of, 223–225

Bisphosphonate-related osteonecrosis of jaws (BRONJ), 228–231
  causes of, 229–230
  clinical presentation of, 228–229
  described, 228
  staging of, 229
  treatment of, 230–231
BMES. See *Bone marrow edema syndrome (BMES).*
BMU. See *Basic multicellular unit (BMU).*
Bone densitometry, in osteonecrosis treatment evaluation, 186
Bone grafting, for secondary osteonecrosis of knee, 205–206
Bone impaction grafting (BIG), THA after, for osteonecrosis of femoral head, 292–293
Bone marrow edema syndrome (BMES)
  characteristics of, 245
  in postpartal women, treatment of, iloprost in, **241–247.** See also *Iloprost, for BMES in postpartal women.*
  pathogenesis of, 241
Bone perfusion, assessment of, contrast-enhanced MRI in, **249–257**
  study of
    discussion of, 251–256
    methods in, 250–251
    results of, 251
Bone remodeling, 213–214
BRONJ. See *Bisphosphonate-related osteonecrosis of jaws (BRONJ).*

C

Cellular-based therapy, for osteonecrosis, **213–221.** See also *Osteonecrosis, treatment of, cellular-based therapy.*
Clinical improvement, biologic improvement vs., in osteonecrosis treatment, 179
Clinical performance, as outcome measure in osteonecrosis treatment evaluation, 179–185
Collapsed SSFFH, **259–265.** See also *Subchondral stress fracture of femoral head (SSFFH), collapsed.*
Composite scoring systems, as outcome measure in osteonecrosis treatment evaluation, 181
Contrast-enhanced MRI, in bone perfusion assessment, **249–257.** See also *Bone perfusion, assessment of, contrast-enhanced MRI in.*
Core decompression
  for secondary osteonecrosis of knee, 205
  for SPONK, 200–201

orthopedic.theclinics.com

Core (*continued*)
with arthroscopic assistance, for secondary
osteonecrosis of knee, 205

D

DCE-MRI, in bone perfusion assessment, 249
Decompression, core. See *Core decompression.*
Densitometry, bone, in osteonecrosis treatment
evaluation, 186
Doppler ultrasonography, in osteonecrosis treatment
evaluation, 186
Dynamic contrast-enhanced MRI (DCE-MRI), in bone
perfusion assessment, 249

F

Femoral head, osteonecrosis of. See *Osteonecrosis,
of femoral head.*
Femoral stems, uncemented primary, for femoral
head osteonecrosis, outcome of, **283–289.** See
also *Uncemented primary femoral stems, for
osteonecrosis of femoral head.*
Function, as outcome measure in osteonecrosis
treatment evaluation, 180

G

Gadolinium-enhanced MRI, in osteonecrosis
treatment evaluation, 186

H

Hemi-resurfacing arthroplasty, for osteonecrosis of
hip, 27-year experience with, **275–282.** See also
*Hip(s), osteonecrosis of, hemi-resurfacing
arthroplasty for, 27-year experience with.*
Hip(s), osteonecrosis of, hemi-resurfacing
arthroplasty for, 27-year experience with, **275–282**
complications in, 278
discussion of, 279–281
indications for, 276
materials and methods in, 275–277
results of, 277–279
revisions in, 278
statistical analysis in, 277
surgical technique, 276–277
survivorship in, 278–279

I

Iloprost, for BMES in postpartal women, **241–247**
study of, 241–246
clinical course of, 242
discussion of, 242–246

materials and methods in, 241–242
MRI follow-up in, 242
participants' characteristics in, 242
results of, 242
side effects of, 242
Imaging, in osteonecrosis treatment evaluation,
185–187

J

Jaw(s), osteonecrosis of, 228
bisphosphonate-related, 228–231. See also
*Bisphosphonate-related osteonecrosis of jaws
(BRONJ).*

K

Knee(s), osteonecrosis of, **193–211**
causes of, 193
conditions associated with, 193. See also *specific
condition, e.g., Spontaneous osteonecrosis of
the knee (SPONK).*
comparison among, 194
incidence of, 193
staging systems for, 196

M

Magnetic resonance imaging (MRI)
contrast-enhanced, in bone perfusion
assessment, **249–257.** See also *Bone
perfusion, assessment of, contrast-enhanced
MRI in.*
gadolinium-enhanced, in osteonecrosis treatment
evaluation, 186
Medical knowledge, defined, 299
Mevalonate pathway, 225
MRI. See *Magnetic resonance imaging (MRI).*

N

Near infrared spectroscopy (NIRS), in osteonecrosis
treatment evaluation, 186–187
NIRS. See *Near infrared spectroscopy (NIRS).*

O

OITE. See *Orthopaedic In-Training Examination
(OITE).*
Orthopaedic In-Training Examination (OITE), recent
literature as tool for learning more about
osteonecrosis in preparation for, study of,
299–304
methods in, 300

purpose of, 299
results of, 300–301
Osteoarthritis, pathophysiology of, 249
Osteochondral defect repair, for SPONK, 200
Osteonecrosis
    bisphosphonates and, **223–234.** See also
        *Bisphosphonate(s); Bisphosphonate-related
        osteonecrosis of jaws (BRONJ).*
    causes of, 227
    characteristics of, 245
    corticosteroid-related, in renal transplant patients,
        study of statin usage effects on, **235–239**
        demographics in, 236
        design of, 235–236
        discussion of, 237–238
        materials and methods in, 235–236
        power analysis in, 236
        results of, 237
        statistical analysis in, 236
    described, 214
    of femoral head
        age as factor in, 267
        bisphosphonates for, 226–228
        failed treatment of, THA after, study of,
            291–298. See also *Total hip arthroplasty
            (THA), after failed treatment for
            osteonecrosis of femoral head, study of.*
        treatment of, cellular-based therapy, 217–218
        TRO for, **291–298.** See also *Transtrochanteric
            rotational osteotomy (TRO), for
            osteonecrosis of femoral head, study of.*
        uncemented primary femoral stems for,
            outcome of, **283–289.** See also
            *Uncemented primary femoral stems, for
            osteonecrosis of femoral head.*
    of hip, hemi-resurfacing arthroplasty for, 27-year
        experience with, **275–282.** See also *Hip(s),
        osteonecrosis of, hemi-resurfacing arthroplasty
        for, 27-year experience with.*
    of knee, **193–211.** See also *Knee(s), osteonecrosis
        of.*
    recent literature as source of information about, in
        OITE preparation, **299–304.** See also
        *Orthopaedic In-Training Examination (OITE),
        recent literature as source of information about
        osteonecrosis in preparation for, study of.*
    treatment of
        bone remodeling in, 213–214
        cellular-based therapy, **213–221**
            marrow cell implantation in, efficacy of, 218
            stem cells in, 215–217
                adult, 214–215
                in bone repair, 215–216
                in vascular repair, 216–217
        clinical improvement vs. biologic improvement
            in, 179
        evaluation of

    biomarkers in, 187
    outcome measures for, **179–191**
        clinical performance, 179–185
        complications, 185
        composite scoring systems, 181
        for biological assessment, 185–187
        function, 180
        imaging in, 185–187
        instruments, 180
        pain relief, 180
        quality of life, 181
        radiographic progression, 181
        selection of, 185
        surgery vs. need for surgery, 181, 185
    outcome measures in, risks–benefits, 185
    studies in, 182–184
Osteotomy
    high tibial, for SPONK, 201
    posterior rotational, high-degree, respherical
        contour with medial collapsed femoral head
        necrosis, in young patients with extensive
        necrosis, **267–274.** See also *Respherical
        contour with medial collapsed femoral head
        necrosis.*
    transtrochanteric rotational, for osteonecrosis of
        femoral head, **291–298**
        study of. See also *Transtrochanteric rotational
            osteotomy (TRO), for osteonecrosis of
            femoral head, study of.*

P

Pain relief, as outcome measure in osteonecrosis
    treatment evaluation, 180
PET. See *Positron emission tomography (PET).*
Positron emission tomography (PET), in
    osteonecrosis treatment evaluation, 187
Postarthroscopic osteonecrosis of knee
    causes of, 206–207
    described, 206
    diagnosis of, 207
    pathogenesis of, 206–207
    pathology of, 206–207
    treatment of, 207–209
        arthroplasty, 207–209
        described, 207
        joint-preserving surgical treatment, 207
        nonoperative, 207
Posterior rotational osteotomy, high-degree,
    respherical contour with medial collapsed femoral
    head necrosis, in young patients with extensive
    necrosis, **267–274.** See also *Respherical contour
    with medial collapsed femoral head necrosis.*
Postpartum women, BMES in, treatment of, iloprost
    in, **241–247.** See also *Iloprost, for BMES in
    postpartal women.*
Pyrophosphate(s), structure of, 223

Q

Quality of life, as outcome measure in osteonecrosis treatment evaluation, 181

R

Radiographic progression, as outcome measure in osteonecrosis treatment evaluation, 181
Renal transplant patients, corticosteroid-related osteonecrosis in, study of statin usage effects on, **235–239**. See also *Osteonecrosis, corticosteroid-related, in renal transplant patients, study of statin usage effects on.*
Respherical contour with medial collapsed femoral head necrosis, after high-degree posterior rotational osteotomy in young patients with extensive necrosis, **267–274**
  study of
    discussion of, 273
    materials and methods in, 268–272
    results of, 272–273

S

Secondary osteonecrosis of knee
  causes of, 202–203
  described, 202
  diagnosis of, 203
  pathogenesis of, 202–203
  pathology of, 202–203
  presentation of, 193
  treatment of, 203–206
    bone grafting, 205–206
    core decompression, 205
      with arthroscopic assistance, 205
    described, 203
    nonoperative, 203–204
    TKA, 206
Spectroscopy
  near infrared, in osteonecrosis treatment evaluation, 186–187
  positron emission, in osteonecrosis treatment evaluation, 187
SPONK. See *Spontaneous osteonecrosis of knee (SPONK).*
Spontaneous osteonecrosis of knee (SPONK)
  causes of, 194–195
  described, 193
  diagnosis of, 195–197
  pathogenesis of, 194–195
  pathology of, 194–195
  presentation of, 193
  treatment of, 197–202

arthroscopy, 199–200
core decompression, 200–201
described, 197–198
high tibial osteotomy, 201
nonoperative, 198–199
osteochondral defect repair, 200
TKA, 202
unilateral knee arthroplasty, 201–202
SSFFH. See *Subchondral stress fracture of femoral head (SSFFH).*
Statin(s), effects on corticosteroid-related osteonecrosis in renal transplant patients, study of, **235–239**. See also *Osteonecrosis, corticosteroid-related, in renal transplant patients, study of statin usage effects on.*
Stem(s), femoral, uncemented primary, for femoral head osteonecrosis, outcome of, **283–289**. See also *Uncemented primary femoral stems, for osteonecrosis of femoral head.*
Stem cells, adult, in osteonecrosis treatment, 214–215
Subchondral stress fracture of femoral head (SSFFH), collapsed, **259–265**
  described, 259
  study of
    discussion of, 264
    materials and methods in, 259–262
    results of, 262–263

T

THA. See *Total hip arthroplasty (THA).*
TKA. See *Total knee arthroplasty (TKA).*
Total hip arthroplasty (THA)
  after BIG, for osteonecrosis of femoral head, 292–293
  after failed treatment for osteonecrosis of femoral head, study of, **291–298**
    discussion of, 294–296
    materials and methods in, 292–293
    radiology in, 294
    results of, 293–294
    statistical analysis in, 293
  after TRO, for osteonecrosis of femoral head, 292
Total knee arthroplasty (TKA)
  for secondary osteonecrosis of the knee, 206
  for SPONK, 202
Transtrochanteric rotational osteotomy (TRO), for osteonecrosis of femoral head
  after failed treatment, study of, **291–298**
    discussion of, 294–296
    materials and methods in, 292–293
    radiology in, 294
    results of, 293–294
THA after, 292

TRO. See *Transtrochanteric rotational osteotomy (TRO)*.

U

Ultrasonography, Doppler, in osteonecrosis treatment evaluation, 186
Uncemented primary femoral stems, for osteonecrosis of femoral head, **283–289**
study of

data collection and analysis in, 286
demographics in, 283–285
discussion of, 287–288
follow-up care in, 286
materials and methods in, 283–286
results of, 286–287
stems in, 285
surgical procedure in, 286
Unilateral knee arthroplasty, for SPONK, 201–202

Moving?

Make sure your subscription moves with you!

To notify us of your new address, find your **Clinics Account Number** (located on your mailing label above your name), and contact customer service at:

E-mail: elspcs@elsevier.com

800-654-2452 (subscribers in the U.S. & Canada)
314-453-7041 (subscribers outside of the U.S. & Canada)

Fax number: 314-523-5170

Elsevier Periodicals Customer Service
11830 Westline Industrial Drive
St. Louis, MO 63146

*To ensure uninterrupted delivery of your subscription, please notify us at least 4 weeks in advance of move.

Printed and bound by CPI Group (UK) Ltd, Croydon, CR0 4YY

03/10/2024

01040352-0015